Evidence-Based Dentistry

Evidenz-basierte Medizin
in der Zahn-, Mund- und Kieferheilkunde

Materialienreihe
Band 23

Winfried Walther, Wolfgang Micheelis
(Gesamtbearbeitung)

Evidence-Based Dentistry

Evidenz-basierte Medizin in der Zahn-, Mund- und Kieferheilkunde

Mit Beiträgen von:
Peter Boehme, Michael Heners, Jörg Michael Herrmann,
Thomas Kerschbaum, Jörg Meyle, Matthias Perleth, Elmar Reich,
Derek Richards, Thure von Uexküll, Wilfried Wagner, Winfried Walther

Herausgeber:
INSTITUT DER DEUTSCHEN ZAHNÄRZTE (IDZ)
in Trägerschaft von
Bundeszahnärztekammer
– Arbeitsgemeinschaft der Deutschen Zahnärztekammern e.V. –
Kassenzahnärztliche Bundesvereinigung – Körperschaft des öffentl. Rechts –
50931 Köln, Universitätsstraße 71–73

Deutscher Zahnärzte Verlag DÄV-Hanser
Köln München 2000

Gesamtbearbeitung:

Prof. Dr. Winfried Walther/Karlsruhe
Dr. Wolfgang Micheelis/Köln

Lektorat/Redaktion:

Dorothee Fink/Köln

Übersetzungen:

Philip Slotkin, M.A. Cantab. M.I.T.I.
London

Dorothee Fink/Köln
(Deutsche Übersetzung Kapitel 2)

Die Deutsche Bibliothek – CIP-Einheitsaufnahme

Evidence-based dentistry : evidenz-basierte Medizin in der Zahn-, Mund- und Kieferheilkunde / Hrsg.: Institut der Deutschen Zahnärzte (IDZ). Winfried Walther ; Wolfgang Micheelis (Gesamtbearb.). Mit Beitr. von: Peter Boehme ... [Übers.: Philipp Slotkin ; Dorothee Fink]. – Köln; München : Dt. Zahnärzte-Verl. DÄV-Hanser, 2000
 (Materialienreihe / Institut der Deutschen Zahnärzte ; Bd. 23)
 ISBN 3-934280-18-8

ISBN 3-934280-18-8

Das Werk ist urheberrechtlich geschützt. Jede Verwertung in anderen als den gesetzlich zugelassenen Fällen bedarf deshalb der vorherigen schriftlichen Genehmigung des Verlages.

Copyright © by Deutscher Zahnärzte Verlag DÄV-Hanser
Köln München 2000

"If a man will begin with certainties, he shall end in doubts; but if he will be content to begin with doubts, he shall end in certainties."

Francis Bacon in *"The Advancement of Learning" (1605)*

Inhaltsverzeichnis / Table of Contents

Geleitwort 13
Foreword 15

Einführung 17
Winfried Walther und *Wolfgang Micheelis*
Introduction 21

1   Die Wissenschaftlichkeit in der Zahnheilkunde 25
Michael Heners

1.1 Vorbemerkung 25
1.2 Aufgabenstellung zahnmedizinischer Wissenschaft 26
1.3 Galileisches Erkenntnisprinzip und reduktionistisches Denken . . 27
1.4 Diskrepanz zwischen ärztlichem Handeln und
     wissenschaftlicher Abstraktion 28
1.5 Paradigmenwechsel in der Zahnheilkunde:
     Herausforderungen einer evidenz-basierten Zahnheilkunde 30

1   Dentistry as a scientific discipline 33
1.1 Preliminary note 33
1.2 Task of dental science 34
1.3 The Galilean epistemological principle and
     reductionistic thinking 34
1.4 Discrepancy between medical activity and scientific abstraction . 36
1.5 Paradigm shift in dentistry: challenges of an evidence-based
     dentistry 38
1.6 *Literatur/References* 40

**2   Entscheidungsfindung auf der Grundlage der besten
     externen wissenschaftlichen Evidenz: Eine Herausforderung
     für den Wissenschaftler und den Praktiker** 41
Derek Richards

2.1 Einleitung 41
2.2 Warum sind Veränderungen erforderlich? 42
2.3 Probleme bei der Umsetzung von Innovationen 42

2.4	Evidenzgrade	44
2.5	Evidenz-Basis in der Zahnheilkunde	45
2.6	Forschung und Anwendung in der evidenz-basierten Zahnheilkunde	48
2.7	Welche Herausforderungen stehen für die Zukunft an?	49
2.8	Die Verbreitung evidenz-basierter Erkenntnisse und Implementationsstrategien	49
2.9	Ausblick	50

2	**Use of best evidence in making decisions: a challenge for the scientist and practitioner**	**53**
2.1	Introduction	53
2.2	Drivers for change	54
2.3	Innovation bypass	54
2.4	Levels of evidence	56
2.5	Dental evidence base	56
2.6	Users and doers	59
2.7	The challenges ahead	60
2.8	Dissemination and implementation	61
2.9	Conclusion	61
2.10	*Literatur/References*	63

3	**Evidenz-basierte Medizin – die Suche und Anwendung von gesicherten Entscheidungsgrundlagen**	**65**
	Matthias Perleth	
3.1	Einleitung: Anmerkungen zum Evidenzbegriff	65
3.2	Was versteht man unter „gesicherter Evidenz"?	66
3.3	Die Cochrane Collaboration	69
3.4	Das Problem der Generalisierbarkeit	69
3.5	Quellen für systematische Übersichten	72
3.6	Anwendungskontext und Ausblick	73

3	**Evidence-based medicine: seeking and applying reliable foundations for decision-making**	**75**
3.1	Introduction: Notes on the concept of evidence	75
3.2	What is meant by "reliable evidence"?	76
3.3	The Cochrane Collaboration	79
3.4	The problem of generalizability	79
3.5	Sources for systematic reviews	82
3.6	Utilization context and outlook	83
3.7	*Literatur/References*	85

4	**Evidenz-basierte und patientenorientierte Medizin – zwei Modelle und ihr Zusammenhang** 87

Jörg Michael Herrmann und Thure von Uexküll

4.1	Vorbemerkung: Zwei Begriffe, viele Fragen, wenig befriedigende Antworten 87
4.2	Das wirkliche Anliegen der neuen Bewegung 88
4.3	Der „Goldstandard" ist inflationär: Widersprüche von EBM 89
4.4	Was ist Evidenz? 90
4.5	Pragmatische und kommunikative Evidenz 91
4.6	Die wissenschaftstheoretische Situation im 20. Jahrhundert 93

4	**Evidence-based and patient-oriented medicine: two models and how they are connected** 95
4.1	Preliminary note: two terms, many questions and few satisfactory answers 95
4.2	The true intent of the new movement 96
4.3	The "gold standard" is inflationary: contradictions of EBM 97
4.4	What is evidence? 98
4.5	Pragmatic and communicative evidence 99
4.6	The epistemological situation in the twentieth century 100
4.7	*Literatur/References* 102

5	**Evidenz-basierte Medizin und die Systematik der klinischen Entscheidungsfindung** 103

Winfried Walther

5.1	Einleitung 103
5.2	Welche Entscheidungsschritte sind Grundlage der systematischen Therapiefindung? Modelle der klinischen Entscheidungsfindung 104
5.3	Wie wird die Therapieentscheidung empirisch gesichert? 109
5.4	Welche Bedeutung hat evidenz-basierte Zahnheilkunde für eine empirisch gesicherte Therapieentscheidung? 112
5.5	Was sind die Merkmale der adäquaten Therapieentscheidung? . 114

5	**Evidence-based medicine and the systematics of clinical decision-making** 117
5.1	Introduction 117
5.2	What decision-making steps underlie systematic determination of the appropriate therapy? Models of clinical decision-making . 118
5.3	How is the decision on therapy underpinned empirically? 122
5.4	What is the significance of evidence-based dentistry for an empirically underpinned therapeutic decision? 126
5.5	What are the characteristics of appropriate decision-making on therapy? 128
5.6	*Literatur/References* 129

6 Evidenz-basierte Zahnheilkunde als Grundlage der prothetischen Therapie 131
Thomas Kerschbaum

- 6.1 Vorbemerkung 131
- 6.2 Warum evidenz-basierte Entscheidungen? 131
- 6.3 Quellen der Evidenz in der Prothetik 134
- 6.4 Problematik prothetischer Leitlinienentwicklung 139
- 6.5 Zusammenfassung 142

6 Evidence-based dentistry as a basis of prosthetic therapy ... 143
- 6.1 Preliminary note 143
- 6.2 Why evidence-based decisions? 143
- 6.3 Sources of evidence in prosthetics 146
- 6.4 Development of prosthetic guidelines: the problems 151
- 6.5 Summary 154
- 6.6 *Literatur/References* 155

7 Evidenz-basierte Zahnheilkunde in der Kariestherapie 159
Elmar Reich

- 7.1 Vorbemerkung 159
- 7.2 Evidenz in der Kariesdiagnose 160
- 7.3 Evidenz in der Prävention 162
- 7.4 Evidenz in der Therapie 165
- 7.5 Kosteneffektivität der Versorgung 168
- 7.6 Ausblick 169

7 Evidence-based dentistry in caries therapy 171
- 7.1 Preliminary note 171
- 7.2 Evidence in caries diagnosis 172
- 7.3 Evidence in prevention 174
- 7.4 Evidence in therapy 176
- 7.5 Cost-effectiveness of treatment 178
- 7.6 Outlook 181
- 7.7 *Literatur/References* 182

8 Evidenz-basierte Konzepte in der parodontologischen Praxis 187
Jörg Meyle

- 8.1 Einleitung 187
- 8.2 Diagnostik und Initialtherapie 187
- 8.3 Weiterführende (chirurgische) Therapie 189
- 8.4 Zusammenfassung 191

8	**Evidence-based approaches to periodontal practice**	193
8.1	Introduction	193
8.2	Diagnosis and initial therapy	193
8.3	Additional (surgical) treatment	195
8.4	Conclusion	196
8.5	*Literatur/References*	198

9	**Brauchen wir neue Forschungsstrategien in der Zahn-, Mund- und Kieferheilkunde?**	201
	Wilfried Wagner	
9.1	Einleitung	201
9.2	Definition und methodische Begrenzung	201
9.3	Notwendigkeit von EBM-Kriterien in Abhängigkeit der Wirksamkeit	203
9.4	Gefahren von EBM-Kriterien	203
9.5	Rückwirkung der EBM auf die Forschung	204
9.6	Veränderungen in der zahnmedizinischen Forschung durch EBM-Strategien	205
9.7	Detailprobleme randomisierter Studien in der Zahnheilkunde	207
9.8	Bedeutung der EBM für die zahnärztliche Qualitätssicherung	209
9.9	Ausblick	210

9	**Do we need new research strategies in dentistry and oral medicine?**	211
9.1	Introduction	211
9.2	Definition and methodological differentiation	211
9.3	Need for EBM criteria in relation to efficacy	213
9.4	Dangers of EBM criteria	213
9.5	Feedback effects of EBM on research	214
9.6	Changes in dental research due to EBM strategies	215
9.7	Detailed problems of randomized studies in dentistry	217
9.8	Importance of EBM for quality assurance	218
9.9	Outlook	219
9.10	*Literatur/References*	220

10	**EBM-Konzepte aus standespolitischer Sicht der Bundeszahnärztekammer – Anforderungen und Folgerungen**	221
	Peter Boehme	

| 10 | EBM concepts from the point of view of the profession as represented by the Bundeszahnärztekammer [German Dental Association] – requirements and conclusions | 227 |

| 11 | Verzeichnis der Autoren | 233 |
| 11 | List of Contributors | 233 |

| 12 | Verzeichnis der Abbildungen und Tabellen | 235 |
| 12 | List of Figures and Tables | 237 |

Geleitwort

Der Gemeinsame Vorstandsausschuss von Bundeszahnärztekammer und Kassenzahnärztlicher Bundesvereinigung für unser Institut der Deutschen Zahnärzte (IDZ) hat das Angebot der angesehenen Akademie für Zahnärztliche Fortbildung/Karlsruhe sehr dankbar aufgenommen, eine gemeinsame Veranstaltung zum Themenkomplex „Evidence-based Dentistry" (EBD) in den Räumlichkeiten und vor allem mit dem großen wissenschaftlichen Know-how der Karlsruher Kollegen durchzuführen.

Die Realisierung einer solchen Veranstaltung zu der Gesamtthematik der „Evidence-Based Medicine" (EBM) war sicherlich schon fast überfällig, um den Stand der Dinge, die Problemstellungen und Perspektiven einer evidenz-basierten Medizin auf dem Gebiet der Zahnheilkunde mit Wissenschaftlern und Vertretern der Gesundheits- und Sozialpolitik in einer gemeinsamen Diskussionsveranstaltung für Deutschland aufzuarbeiten.

„Überfällig" auch deswegen, weil sich die großen forschungspolitischen Entwicklungslinien zu EBM sowohl im internationalen als auch im nationalen Rahmen zunehmend mit ökonomischen und fiskalischen Fragen und Erwartungen zur politischen Steuerung der Gesundheitssysteme verbinden und es von daher einer ausreichenden Abklärung bedarf, was EBM bzw. EBD kann und was EBM bzw. EBD nicht kann: Denn Fragen einer evidenzbasierten Ausübung der Zahnheilkunde im Versorgungsalltag sind eo ipso nicht mit Fragen von Kosteneinsparungen bei zahnärztlichen Dienstleistungen gleichzusetzen; der Zusammenhang zwischen beiden Parametern erscheint uns sehr viel komplizierter zu sein! Wir sind deswegen sehr froh, dass es durch die hervorragenden Referenten im Rahmen dieser Veranstaltung gelungen ist, die Vielschichtigkeit von EBM bzw. EBD deutlich zu machen und auch ungelöste Fragen auf diesem Gebiet offen anzusprechen.

An den Chancen, die sich mit einer stärkeren Evidenzbasierung ärztlicher/zahnärztlicher Dienstleistungen verbinden, kann unserer Auffassung nach allerdings auch kein Zweifel bestehen: Angesichts der rasanten wissenschaftlichen Entwicklung kann sie dazu beitragen, dass gesicherte Erkenntnisse systematisch und schneller in die Versorgung Eingang finden. Zweifellos wird ein enger „Schulterschluss" zwischen Wissenschaft und Praxis das Anliegen einer zahnmedizinischen Qualitätssicherung für die diagnostischen bzw. therapeutischen Methoden auf eine noch bessere Basis stellen.

Wir danken an dieser Stelle sehr herzlich allen Beteiligten bei der Ausrichtung dieses Symposiums und wünschen dem nunmehr vorgelegten Reader in der IDZ-Materialienreihe einen hoffentlich großen Leserkreis. Die deutsch-englische Herausgabe der Texte wird sicherlich helfen, den internationalen Austausch gerade auf dem Gebiet der Evidence-based Dentistry zu befruchten.

Dr. Fritz-Josef Willmes
(Amtierender Vorsitzender
des Gemeinsamen
IDZ-Vorstandsausschusses)

Dr. Karl Horst Schirbort
(Alternierender Vorsitzender
des Gemeinsamen
IDZ-Vorstandsausschusses)

Köln, im Februar 2000

Foreword

The Joint Executive Committee of our Institute of German Dentists (IDZ), comprising representatives of the German Dental Association (BZÄK) and the Federal Authority for Dental Care (KZBV), has gratefully accepted the offer of the respected Academy for Postgraduate Dental Studies, Karlsruhe, to hold a joint symposium on the various aspects of evidence-based dentistry (EBD) on the premises of our Karlsruhe colleagues, where we were able, in particular, to benefit from their high-level scientific know-how.

It was surely high time to hold a meeting of this kind on the entire field of evidence-based medicine (EBM), bringing together on a joint discussion platform both scientists and makers of health and social policy in Germany to assess the situation, issues and prospects of an evidence-based form of medicine in the sphere of dentistry.

Another reason why such an event was overdue is that the major lines of development in EBM research are increasingly bound up, both nationally and internationally, with economic and fiscal questions and expectations concerning the political control of health systems, so that it is essential to clarify adequately what EBM/EBD can and cannot do. After all, the evidence-based practice of dentistry in a routine treatment setting cannot automatically be equated with the aim of cutting the cost of dental services; the connection between the two parameters seems to us to be much more complicated than that! We are therefore very pleased that the eminent contributors to this symposium have succeeded both in demonstrating the full complexity of EBM/EBD and in openly addressing some of the unresolved problems in this field.

Nor, in our view, can there be any doubt about the potential benefits of a firmer basis of evidence for medical and dental services: considering the enormous pace of scientific development, such an approach can help to ensure the prompt and systematic transfer of new, reliably based knowledge and discoveries to the practical treatment situation. If science and dental practice stand shoulder to shoulder in this way, the aim of placing dental quality assurance for diagnostic and therapeutic methods on an even sounder foundation will be well served.

We should like to take this opportunity of thanking all those involved in the organization of this symposium, and trust that the documentation here presented in the IDZ publication series will enjoy a wide readership. Its bilingual publication in German and English will surely prove fruitful in facilitating international exchanges precisely in the field of evidence-based dentistry.

Dr. Fritz-Josef Willmes
(Acting Chairman of the
IDZ Joint Executive Committee)

Dr. Karl Horst Schirbort
(Rotating Chairman of the
IDZ Joint Executive Committee)

Cologne, February 2000

Einführung

Winfried Walther, Karlsruhe
Wolfgang Micheelis, Köln

Die Anforderungen an die zahnärztliche Praxis sind in den letzten Jahren erheblich gestiegen. Der praktizierende Zahnarzt spürt dies durch die gewachsenen Erwartungen seiner Patienten und durch die gesellschaftliche Diskussion über die ärztliche Tätigkeit. So hat die Forderung nach Qualitätssicherung in der Medizin bereits vor Jahren ärztliche und zahnärztliche Handlungsroutinen in Frage gestellt. Seit „Evidence-based Medicine" von den Medien als Schlagwort aufgenommen wurde und in der politischen Diskussion Bedeutung errang, sind Ärzte und Zahnärzte mit einer neuen Anforderung konfrontiert, die diesmal auf die Grundlagen der ärztlichen Entscheidungsfindung zielt. Ausgangspunkt der EBM-Diskussion war die Forderung:

– Wichtiges Wissen über die Eignung therapeutischer und diagnostischer Maßnahmen muss in der Praxis ankommen.
– Das gesicherte Wissen muss das weniger gesicherte Wissen ablösen.

Neue Anforderungen sind unbequem. Sie zwingen zur Inventur des Vertrauten und zur Prüfung der Handlungsroutinen. Möglicherweise sind sie die Initialzündung für neue Konzepte, sie können jedoch auch, wenn sie sich als nicht sachgemäß erweisen, Verwirrung und Abwehr auslösen.

Arzt sowie Zahnarzt arbeiten in einem sehr empfindlichen Bereich, der durch das Vertrauen zwischen Behandler und Patient bestimmt und eingegrenzt wird. Es ist deswegen nicht sinnvoll, dem Arzt neue Begriffe ohne praktische Prüfung ihres Inhalts anzupreisen. Auch die Begrifflichkeit der „Evidence-based Medicine" bedarf der Prüfung und der geschulten Interpretation, bevor ihr Platz in der medizinischen Praxis bestimmt werden kann. Aus diesem Grunde entstand der Plan, ein gemeinsames Symposium der Akademie für Zahnärztliche Fortbildung Karlsruhe und des Instituts der Deutschen Zahnärzte/Köln durchzuführen. Ziel der Veranstaltung war, dieses neue Feld der wissenschaftlichen Prüfung von Handlungswissen von verschiedenen kompetenten Referenten darstellen zu lassen und seine Umsetzbarkeit zu untersuchen.

Das Symposium wurde als 7. Karlsruher Expertengespräch und als 10. IDZ-Symposium von den tragenden Institutionen als Gemeinschaftsprojekt am 8. Dezember 1999 in Karlsruhe ausgerichtet. Wir freuen uns, dass es mit den vereinten Kräften aller Beteiligten gelungen ist, nunmehr einer breiteren Öffentlichkeit eine schriftliche Dokumentation dieser Veranstaltung zu „Evidence-based Dentistry (EBD)" in der IDZ-Materialienreihe vorlegen zu können.

Insgesamt waren zu diesem EBD-Symposium rund 100 geladene Gäste aus der zahnmedizinischen Wissenschaft, der zahnärztlichen Standespolitik, den gesetzlichen Krankenkassen, dem Bundesministerium für Gesundheit, dem gesundheits- und sozialpolitischen Journalismus und natürlich auch interessierte Einzelpersonen aus Wissenschaft und Praxis zugegen. Man hatte Gelegenheit, mit den vortragenden Referenten die Fragestellungen, offenen Probleme und Perspektiven von Evidence-based Medicine bzw. Evidence-based Dentistry unter den Rahmenbedingungen des deutschen Ausbildungs- und Versorgungssystems im Medizinbereich zu diskutieren.

Die Referenten rekrutierten sich aus der zahnmedizinischen Wissenschaft, einem Mediziner mit Public Health-Ausrichtung und einem medizinischen Vertreter der psychotherapeutischen Medizin. Ein standespolitischer Referent der Bundeszahnärztekammer rundete diesen Referentenkreis ab.

Die Dokumentation stellt eine vollständige Übersicht über alle im Verlaufe des EBD-Symposiums gehaltenen Referate her; alle Referenten waren zu diesem Zweck gebeten worden, ihre mündlichen Ausführungen in Schriftform zu bringen und bei Bedarf auch noch redaktionell zu bearbeiten. Insbesondere galt das Augenmerk einer detaillierten Dokumentation der in den Referaten verarbeiteten bzw. zitierten Literatur.

Um der vorgelegten IDZ-Publikation auch im angloamerikanischen Sprachraum eine Chance zur Kommunikation zu geben, wurden alle Referententexte zusätzlich ins Englische (bzw. im Falle von Herrn Richards ins Deutsche) übersetzt. Wir glauben, dass damit gerade auch dem Anliegen der Evidence-based Medicine im Sinne eines internationalen Austauschs und internationaler Verständigung ein Stück weit Rechnung getragen wurde.

In den Diskussionen der Teilnehmer des Symposiums zu den einzelnen Referaten, aber selbstverständlich auch in den Referaten selbst, schälten sich nach unserer Einschätzung drei große Fragegruppen heraus, die sich in Anlehnung an den programmatischen Artikel von Bader, Ismail und Clarkson (1999)[1] vielleicht folgendermaßen zusammenfassen lassen:

---

[1] Bader, J., Ismail, A., Clarkson, J.: Evidence-based dentistry and the dental research community. J Dent Res 78 (9), 1999, 1480–1483

1. Was heißt eigentlich „Evidenz" in der Medizin/Zahnmedizin, und wer produziert diese Evidenz?
2. Wie kann evidenz-basiertes Wissen anwenderorientiert verfügbar gemacht werden?
3. Welche Rolle kann evidenz-basiertes Wissen in der zahnmedizinischen Praxis spielen? Inwieweit ist es nützlich und einsetzbar?

Erwartungsgemäß gab es auf diese drei großen Fragekomplexe keine abschließenden Antworten, da das Thema von EBM bzw. EBD insgesamt noch viel zu jung ist und noch in voller Entwicklungsdynamik steckt; ganz abgesehen davon, dass auf dem Gebiet der Zahnmedizin der EBM-Gedanke erst mit einer gewissen Verspätung eingesetzt hat. Hinzu kommt, dass Evidence-based Medicine/Evidence-based Dentistry insbesondere das komplizierte Verhältnis von Theorie und Praxis noch keineswegs ausreichend ausgeleuchtet hat: Der praktisch-konkrete Umgang mit EBM-Wissensbeständen im ärztlichen Versorgungsalltag gehorcht zweifellos einer eigenständigen Bedingungsstruktur, da naturgemäß nicht Krankheiten, sondern erkrankte Menschen zu versorgen sind. Dies aber bedeutet, dass das evidenz-basierte Wissen durch den Arzt/Zahnarzt gleichsam erst passend gemacht werden muss, um im individuellen Behandlungsfall einsetzbar zu sein; zusätzlich gehen in diesen komplizierten Transformationsprozess Aspekte der Patientenseite im Sinne von subjektiven Präferenzen und Erwartungen ein. Der Begriff der „kommunikativen Evidenz" (siehe hierzu auch Kapitel 4) mag hier die Richtung des Gemeinten fokussieren. Insgesamt muss also auch der Praxis, also auch den Alltagsbedingungen und den Erfahrungen der klinischen Praxis, ein angemessenes Gewicht eingeräumt werden, um dem EBM-Gedanken „Bodenhaftung" zu geben.

Und zweifellos ist auch für das Feld der Evidence-based Dentistry noch unklar, welche methodisch-wissenschaftlichen Stufen der Evidenz realistischerweise favorisiert werden können, da beispielsweise randomisierte klinische Studien (RCTs) sicherlich nicht zu allen diagnostischen und/oder therapeutischen Verfahren aufgelegt werden können bzw. noch nicht einmal unbedingt sinnvoll sind. Darüber hinaus gibt es in der Zahnmedizin – wie selbstverständlich in der Medizin insgesamt – ein Spektrum von Forschungsfragen, die sich mit dem Methodeninstrumentarium von EBM/EBD nicht bearbeiten lassen.

Alles in allem scheinen uns aber die Vorträge und die Diskussionen des Symposiums deutlich gemacht zu haben, dass das Fazit dieser Veranstaltung war, EBD – als Teil von EBM – als eine Chance zu begreifen, das Nachdenken in der Zahnmedizin auf eine neue, methodenbewusstere und methodenkritischere Basis zu stellen. Die Früchte dieses neuen Gedankenansatzes zur systematischen Erschließung von Wissensquellen aus der wissenschaftlichen Forschung kommen aber zweifellos auch der zahnärztlichen Praxis zugute, die dadurch klare Entscheidungshilfen bzw. Entscheidungsunterstützungen erhält; wichtig scheint nur, dass hier der strukturell notwendige Handlungsspielraum (Handlungskorridore) für die alltägliche Versorgungspraxis erhalten bleibt. Und deutlich wurde in der Diskussion auch, dass die Gesundheitspolitik durch EBM/EBD vor völlig neue Herausforderungen und Begründungsdimensionen gestellt wird, da evidenz-basiertes Versorgungshandeln im Gesundheitssystem Fragen von Kosten-Nutzen-Relationen einzelner medizinischer Maßnahmen in völlig neuer Weise aufrollt. Denn natürlich kann die systematische Berücksichtigung evidenzbasierter Wissensbestände beispielsweise bei einer zahnärztlichen Therapieplanung die Therapiekosten verteuern und gerade nicht verbilligen, da die gesicherte Methode nicht zwangsläufig diejenige ist, die weniger Kosten verursacht. EBM bzw. EBD sind jedenfalls kein Instrument kurzfristiger Kostensenkung in der Gesundheitspolitik!

Es ist uns ein Anliegen, an dieser Stelle noch einmal ganz herzlich allen Referenten für ihre interessanten Vorträge zu danken und für die Mühen, die sie mit der Vorbereitung dieser Publikation hatten. Ohne das große und kompetente Engagement der Referenten wäre dieses EBD-Symposium – übrigens das erste seiner Art in Deutschland – nicht möglich gewesen. Ein besonderer Dank gilt Herrn Philip Slotkin, London, der für die englische Übersetzung der Beiträge verantwortlich zeichnet, sowie Herrn Stephen Hancocks, London, für seine Unterstützung und Beratung in Bezug auf die englische Fachterminologie. Schließlich möchten wir uns auch bei Frau Brita Nürnberger von der Akademie für Zahnärztliche Fortbildung/Karlsruhe und Frau Dorothee Fink vom Institut der Deutschen Zahnärzte/Köln bedanken, die durch ihre tatkräftige Mithilfe bei der technischen Organisation des Symposiums viel zum Gelingen beigetragen haben.

Introduction

Winfried Walther, Karlsruhe
Wolfgang Micheelis, Köln

The demands imposed on the practice of dentistry have increased substantially in the last few years. Dental practitioners are aware of this through the increased expectations of their patients on the one hand and the social debate on medical activity on the other. For instance, it is already some years since medical and dental working routines were called into question by the requirement of quality assurance in medicine. Since evidence-based medicine was taken up by the media as a catchphrase and became a political issue, doctors and dentists have been confronted with a new demand, this time directed towards the foundations of medical decision-making. Underlying the EBM debate were the following demands:

— Important knowledge concerning the appropriateness of therapeutic and diagnostic measures must find its way to the practitioner.
— Knowledge underpinned by evidence must take the place of knowledge that lacks this foundation.

New demands are uncomfortable. They force us to take stock of the familiar and to scrutinize our working routines. While they may provide the initial stimulus for new concepts, they may also generate confusion and resistance if they prove impractical.

Doctors and dentists alike work in a very sensitive field, determined and delimited by trust between therapist and patient. It is therefore inappropriate to commend new ideas to practitioners unless their content has been tested in practice. The notions of evidence-based medicine, too, must be subjected to scrutiny and expert interpretation before their place in medical practice can be specified. This was the background to the proposal for the holding of a joint symposium by the Academy for Postgraduate Dental Studies, Karlsruhe, and the Institute of German Dentists, Cologne. Its object was to call upon a group of contributors with differing areas of expertise to introduce this new field of scientific testing of practical know-how and to examine its potential for implementation in practice.

The symposium was held in Karlsruhe on 8 December 1999 as the 7th Karlsruhe Experts' Colloquium and the 10th IDZ Symposium and took the form of a joint project by the sponsoring institutions. We are gratified that, thanks to the united efforts of all concerned, we are now able to present the papers from this meeting on evidence-based dentistry (EBD) to a wider public through the medium of the IDZ publication series.

The EBD symposium brought together in all some 100 invited guests from the fields of dental science, the professional dental organizations, the legal health insurance funds, the Federal Ministry of Health, the health- and social-policy press and also, of course, interested individuals from the spheres of dental science and practice. The opportunity was taken to discuss with the contributors the issues, unresolved problems and prospects of evidence-based medicine and evidence-based dentistry within the framework of the German system of medical education and health care.

The contributors included representatives of academic dentistry, a doctor specializing in public health issues and a medical psychotherapist. Finally, the professional organizations were represented by a contributor from the German Dental Association.

The documentation comprises all the papers presented during the EBD symposium; for this purpose, all contributors were requested to write up their oral presentations and to edit them where necessary. Particular importance was attached to detailed documentation of the literature drawn upon and/or cited in the papers.

To assure this IDZ publication of a wider audience in the English-speaking world, all the German papers have been translated into that language; Dr. Richards's paper appears in a German translation as well as the original English. We believe that this will also help evidence-based medicine to achieve its aim of facilitating international exchanges and understanding.

The interventions from the floor on the individual papers and, of course, the papers themselves seem to us to have centred on three main groups of questions, which can perhaps be summarized as follows in accordance with the criteria set out in the programmatic article by Bader, Ismail & Clarkson (1999)[1]:

1. What does "evidence" actually mean in medicine and dentistry, and who produces this evidence?
2. How can evidence-based knowledge be made available in user-oriented form?
3. What part can evidence-based knowledge play in dental practice? How far is it useful and suitable for practical application?

---

[1] Bader, J., Ismail, A., Clarkson, J.: Evidence-based dentistry and the dental research community. J Dent Res 78 (9), 1999, 1480–1483

As expected, conclusive answers to these three major question complexes were not forthcoming, as EBM/EBD as a whole is still far too young and in the full throes of development – quite apart from the fact that the idea of EBM gained currency in dentistry somewhat later than in other fields. Furthermore, evidence-based medicine/evidence-based dentistry has, in particular, not yet adequately clarified the complicated relationship between theory and practice. The corpus of evidence-based knowledge certainly finds its practical, concrete application in the everyday routine of medical care in a very specific context, because one is treating not diseases but the people suffering from them. However, this means that evidence-based knowledge must as it were first be adapted by the doctor or dentist for use in the treatment of an individual patient; and another factor in this complicated process of transformation will be the patient's subjective preferences and expectations. The notion of "communicative evidence" (cf. chapter 4 in this volume) may help us to understand what is meant here. Overall, therefore, sufficient account must also be taken of the practical environment – that is, of the everyday conditions and experiences of clinical practice – if the notions of EBM are to retain contact with the reality on the ground.

Again, in the field of evidence-based dentistry too, it is surely not yet clear which methodological and scientific levels of evidence can realistically be favoured, considering that, for example, randomized clinical trials (RCTs) cannot of course be stipulated for all diagnostic and therapeutic procedures, nor are they necessarily always appropriate. Furthermore, the discipline of dentistry – as well as, of course, that of medicine as a whole – includes a wide range of research issues that are not amenable to the application of EBM/EBD methods.

All in all, however, the outcome of the symposium's papers and discussions seems to us to be that EBD – as a part of EBM – should be seen as an opportunity to lay new foundations for reflection in dentistry, involving both a greater awareness of our methods and a more critical attitude towards them. This new approach to the systematic utilization of the knowledge accruing from scientific research will certainly bear fruit for the dental practitioner, in the form of clear aids and support for his decision-making – but the freedom of action necessary by virtue of the structure of day-to-day treatment practice must be preserved. The discussion also showed that EBM/EBD imposes novel challenges and dimensions of justification on health policy, because an evidential basis for treatment in the health system poses questions of the cost-benefit ratios of individual medical measures in a wholly new way. After all, systematic allowance for the corpus of evidence-based knowledge may, for example, increase rather than reduce the cost of a dental treatment plan, as the evidence-based method will not necessarily be the cheapest. EBM/EBD is at any rate not an instrument for reducing health-policy costs in the short term!

We should like at this point once again to thank all the contributors warmly for their interesting papers and for their efforts in the preparation of this publication. Without the profound and scholarly commitment of the contributors, this EBD symposium – which is, incidentally, the first of its kind in Germany – would not have been possible. Furthermore, we wish to express our sincere thanks to Philip Slotkin, London, who translated the German papers into English and thus helped us to make this bilingual publication a reality, and to Stephen Hancocks, London, for his kind assistance with specialized terminology. We also owe a particular debt of gratitude to Brita Nürnberger, of the Academy for Postgraduate Dental Studies, Karlsruhe, and Dorothee Fink of the Institute of German Dentists, Cologne, who played a major part in the success of the symposium through their active involvement in its technical organization.

1 Die Wissenschaftlichkeit in der Zahnheilkunde

Michael Heners, Karlsruhe

1.1 Vorbemerkung

Die Zahnheilkunde wird – wie die gesamte Heilkunde – immer stärker von Fragestellungen herausgefordert, die sie zwingen, die Grundlagen für ihr Handeln zu klären. Hierzu gehört auch die Frage nach der wissenschaftlichen Evidenz der zahnärztlichen Entscheidungsgründe. Diese Frage impliziert auch die Frage nach der Wissenschaftlichkeit in der Zahnmedizin.

Dass Zahnheilkunde auf wissenschaftliche Erkenntnisse zu gründen ist, hat in Deutschland der Gesetzgeber erkannt und festgelegt. Im Gesetz über die Ausübung der Zahnheilkunde wird bestimmt: „Zahnheilkunde ist die berufsmäßige, auf zahnärztliche wissenschaftliche Erkenntnisse gegründete Feststellung und Behandlung von Zahn-, Mund- und Kieferkrankheiten. Als Krankheit ist jede von der Norm abweichende Erscheinung im Bereich des Mundes und der Kiefer anzusehen, einschließlich der Anomalien der Zahnstellung und des Fehlens von Zähnen" (vgl. Gesetze für Ärzte und andere Heilberufe, 1995).

Mit diesem Gesetz definierte der Gesetzgeber nicht nur den Tätigkeitsbereich des Zahnarztes – „Feststellung und Behandlung von Zahn-, Mund- und Kieferkrankheiten" –, sondern er legte auch unzweideutig fest, dass diese Tätigkeit berufsmäßig und auf wissenschaftliche Erkenntnisse gegründet sein muss. Was bedeutet also „wissenschaftliche Erkenntnis"?

Wissenschaftliche Erkenntnis wird häufig gleichgesetzt mit Äußerungen, die aus dem formalen Betrieb wissenschaftlicher Einrichtungen resultieren und die durch die Attribute dieser Einrichtungen – z. B. Universität, Akademie, Professor, Doktor, Master of Arts etc. – ihre Autorität erlangen. Hochschulen und Universitäten wurden nun tatsächlich gegründet, um der Wissenschaft einen Raum zur Entfaltung zu geben, sei es durch Forschung und/oder Lehre. Aber gerade die Tatsache, dass alle solchermaßen ideell gegründeten Freiräume auch eines formalen Apparates bedürfen, um funktionsfähig zu sein, bewirkt auch, dass sich zwischen ideeller Aufgabenstellung und formalem Apparat, zwischen ideellem Anspruch und formaler Wirklichkeit Diskrepanzen entwickeln können, die die ursprüngliche Aufgabenstellung verdrängen. Aus solchen Entwicklungen entsteht nicht nur Starrheit, sondern auch neue Orientierung, die wohl immer das gleiche Ziel hat, nämlich, einen in Formalien sich selbst gefallenden Wissenschaftsbetrieb wieder zu seiner ursprünglichen Aufgabenstellung bzw. seinem originären Sinn zurückzuführen. Dazu gehört auch der wissenschaftlich neuartige Gedankenansatz der „Evidence-based Medicine".

1.2 Aufgabenstellung zahnmedizinischer Wissenschaft

Was ist die Aufgabenstellung bzw. der originäre Sinn zahnmedizinischer Wissenschaft? Die Antwort müsste in Anlehnung an das Zahnheilkundegesetz lauten: die Feststellung und Behandlung von Erkrankungen im Zahn-, Mund- und Kieferbereich in ihrer Komplexität und ihrer tatsächlichen Kompliziertheit nachprüfbar zu beschreiben. Da Zahnheilkunde eine zweckbestimmte Wissenschaft ist, geschieht diese Beschreibung nicht um ihrer selbst willen, sondern um den Zahnarzt in die Lage zu versetzen, dem oder der Hilfesuchenden mit nachprüfbaren Methoden zur Seite stehen zu können. Zahnheilkunde ist deshalb – wie die gesamte Heilkunde – sowohl als theoretische als auch als praktische Wissenschaft ohne ethische Basis orientierungslos.

Schließlich muss die Beschreibung der Erkrankungen im Zahn-, Mund- und Kieferbereich nachprüfbar sein. Das bedeutet, die angewandten Methoden zum Erkennen und zur Beschreibung der komplexen zahnärztlichen Vielfalt müssen logischen und eindeutig definierten Regeln folgen. Man nennt dies Methodik der Wissenschaft (vgl. Heners, 1985). Da die Methodik meist recht kompliziert ist und spezifischen Sachverstand erfordert, ist das Erlernen des aus der Anwendung dieser Methodik erworbenen Wissens an ein spezifisches Studium gebunden. Es ist deshalb sinnvoll und ohne Alternative, dass die Ausübung der Zahnheilkunde an ein Studium und die Ausübung wissenschaftlicher Tätigkeit an die die Arbeitsmethoden sichernden Institutionen gebunden ist. Dies gilt zumindest, solange man Zahnheilkunde im modernen Sinne wissenschaftlich begründen und betreiben will.

Heilkundliche Maßnahmen sind immer „Eingriffe". Schipperges (1970) führt dazu aus: „Das spezifische Tun des Arztes besteht darin, dass er, um Hilfe gerufen und um die Not abzuwenden, einzugreifen hat. Der Arzt greift dabei immer in die Integrität des Menschen ein, nicht allein mit dem Messer, sondern auch mit der Droge, er greift ein sogar mit seinem Rat und seiner Ratlosigkeit". Die Ungewissheit ärztlichen Handelns macht es verständlich, dass am Anfang wissenschaftlich betriebener Heilkunde die Bestimmung ihrer ethischen Rahmenbedingungen steht (vgl. Abb. 1-1).

Die im hippokratischen Eid festgelegten Regeln des „Nihil nocere" (Nie schaden) und des „Solus aegroti salus" (Nur der Wohlfahrt des Patienten dienend) limitieren bis zum heutigen Tag ärztliches Handeln (vgl. Ankermann, 1991).

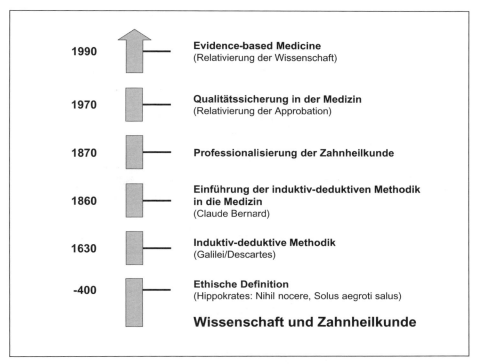

Abbildung 1-1: Etappen in der Wissenschaftlichkeit von Medizin und Zahnheilkunde

1.3 Galileisches Erkenntnisprinzip und reduktionistisches Denken

Die Entdeckung der methodischen Arbeitsweise der modernen Naturwissenschaften, nämlich Verwerfung der Autorität in Fragen wissenschaftlicher Erkenntnis und Gründung allgemeiner Sätze ausschließlich auf Beobachtung und Experiment (Galileo Galilei, sogenanntes induktives Schlussverfahren, vgl. Abb. 1-2), ist für die Wissenschaftlichkeit in der Zahnmedizin insofern von Bedeutung, als Jahrhunderte nach deren Entdeckung 1860 von Claude Bernard diese Arbeitsmethodik auch zur Beschreibung der Gesetzmäßigkeiten von gesundem und erkranktem Körper in die Medizin eingeführt wurde. Diese Arbeitsmethodik ist international bis zum heutigen Tag mehr oder weniger verbindlich für das, was wir Schulmedizin nennen.

Die konsequente und/oder rigorose Anwendung des galileischen Erkenntnisprinzips hat aber nicht nur zu einer enormen und unglaublichen Erweiterung medizinischen Wissens und medizinischer Kunst geführt, sondern sie hat das medizinische Wissen auch unübersehbar werden lassen.

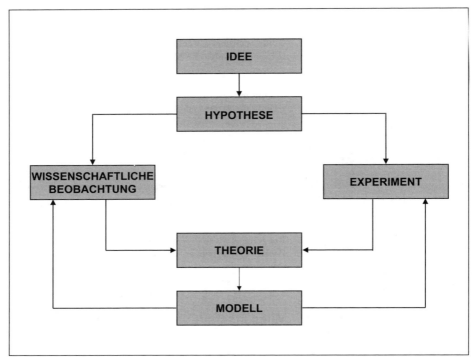

Abbildung 1-2: Das Prinzip der induktiv-deduktiven Erkenntnis

Schließlich konnte diese Methodik nur dann sinnvoll angewendet werden, wenn man sich vorher von der Herausforderung verabschiedete, „das Ganze sehen zu wollen". Dies formulierte René Descartes vor etwa 350 Jahren so: „Wenn ein Problem so komplex ist, dass du es nicht auf einmal lösen kannst, so zerlege es in viele Unterprobleme, die dann entsprechend klein sind, so dass du jedes dieser Unterprobleme lösen kannst". Mit diesem „Reduktionsprinzip" hat die moderne Medizin gelernt, Krankheiten zu erkennen und zu heilen, die sie vor Anwendung dieses Prinzips weder erkennen noch heilen konnte. Aber sie hat auch stillschweigend geschluckt, dass sie den Kranken oder Gesunden „nur reduktionistisch" betrachtet (vgl. Zenner, 2000; Heners, 1977).

1.4 Diskrepanz zwischen ärztlichem Handeln und wissenschaftlicher Abstraktion

Die Fülle der aus dieser Arbeitsmethodik mündenden Informationen stellte zwangsläufig in unserer Zeit zwei Parameter in Frage, die bis dahin unerschütterliche Grundlage ärztlicher Berufsausübung waren: den Absolutheitsanspruch der ärztlichen Approbation und denjenigen der wissenschaft-

1.4 Diskrepanz zwischen ärztlichem Handeln und wissenschaftlicher Abstraktion

lichen Information. Da nämlich ärztliches Handeln nur dann sinnvoll und erfolgreich sein kann, wenn es den Patienten „als Ganzes" einbezieht, lag es auch auf der Hand, nachzufragen, ob die zur Verfügung stehenden Informationen vor Ort, also bei der Behandlung des einzelnen Patienten, zu einer sinnvollen Einheit durch den Arzt zusammengefasst werden. Die Forderung nach „Qualitätssicherung in der Medizin" erscheint deshalb als Versuch, die Kompliziertheit ärztlichen Handelns in das Bewusstsein des Arztes zurückzuholen. Die ärztliche Approbation wird insofern relativiert, als ärztliches Handeln ohne qualitätssichernde Begleitung in Frage gestellt ist.

Die Formulierung der Vorstellungen einer evidenz-basierten Medizin gehen darüber hinaus. Sie stellen die wissenschaftliche Information und die auf ihr basierenden Entscheidungen für ärztliches Handeln selbst in Frage. Dieser Ansatz zielt sowohl auf die medizinische Wissenschaft als auch auf den Praktiker, der ja klinische Probleme lösen muss. Die Wissenschaft soll methodisch in die Pflicht genommen werden, damit die Praxis relevante und unverzerrte Aussagen zur Entscheidung vorfindet. Der Praktiker soll sich seinen eigenen Problemen methodisch nähern und hierbei das beste zur Verfügung stehende Wissen anwenden.

Es wird erkennbar, dass „Wissenschaft" und „ärztliches Handeln" ein Begriffspaar sind, das sich in den vergangenen hundert Jahren gut bewährt hat, dessen Leistungsfähigkeit jedoch an seine Grenzen gestoßen ist und deshalb notwendiger und hoffentlich erfolgreicher Korrekturen bedarf. Ärztliches Handeln ausschließlich „wissenschaftlich" zu begründen, ist nämlich von jeher auf gesunde Skepsis gestoßen. Der britische Internist Sir William Osler formulierte zu Beginn des 20. Jahrhunderts: „The practise of medicine is an art based on science". Er versuchte, mit dieser Formulierung die Diskrepanz zwischen ärztlichem Handeln und wissenschaftlicher Abstraktion darzulegen. Die Parameter, die zahnärztliches Handeln bestimmen, sind in der Abbildung 1-3 zusammengefasst (vgl. Abb. 1-3).

Es wird unterschieden zwischen der Software zahnärztlichen Handelns (das, was man nicht sehen kann) und der Hardware, der klassischen manipulativen Tätigkeit. In Ergänzung zur ärztlichen Tätigkeit in der o. g. Definition von Schipperges zeichnet sich nämlich das spezifisch zahnärztliche Tun dadurch aus, dass der Zahnarzt nicht nur mit dem Messer und der Droge, mit dem Rat und mit der Ratlosigkeit in die Integrität des Menschen eingreift, sondern auch mit seiner restaurativen Kunst. Außerdem vollzieht sich der zahnärztliche Eingriff nicht unsichtbar, sondern stellt sich dem beobachtenden Auge des Patienten. Die Urteilskraft des Zahnarztes, die einem Eingriff vorausgeht und ihn bis zur Vollendung begleitet, findet also ihre Bestätigung oder auch nicht.

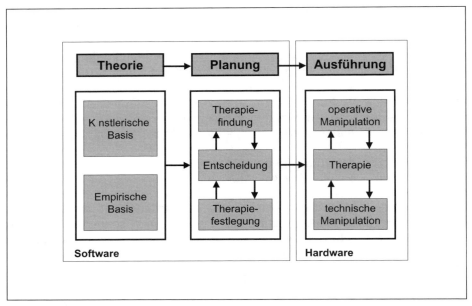

Abbildung 1-3: Parameter der zahnärztlichen Therapie und Therapieentscheidung

1.5 Paradigmenwechsel in der Zahnheilkunde: Herausforderungen einer evidenz-basierten Zahnheilkunde

Dieser Umstand, dass Zahnheilkunde unter dem beobachtenden Auge des Patienten stattfindet, hat das Eigenverständnis der Zahnheilkunde nachhaltig geprägt. Es ist ein Verständnis von Zahnheilkunde, das an anderer Stelle als „Handwerkermodell" bezeichnet wird (vgl. Heners und Walther, 2000). Klassische und bis zum heutigen Tage kritiklos angewandte Entscheidungsparameter dieses Modells sind Banalitäten wie „Wenn man nur immer alles ordentlich macht, kann einem nichts passieren" oder „Das Schönere ist das Bessere", „Das Bessere ist der Feind des Guten" und – sozusagen als Subsummation für wirtschaftliche Erörterungen – „Das Teurere ist das Gesündere!" Das Teuflische an diesen Banalitäten ist – und das gilt ja meist für Banalitäten –, dass sie so plausibel wirken, dass sie scheinbar keiner weiteren Begründung bedürfen. Dennoch treffen sie nicht zu! Diese Banalitäten bestimmen trotzdem weitgehend die fachliche Diskussion in der Zahnheilkunde. Sie sind sozusagen das wissenschaftliche Paradigma, von dem man sich, da es so banal und einfach ist, nicht trennen möchte.

Mit dem Begriff „Paradigma" bezeichnete der Wissenschaftstheoretiker Thomas S. Kuhn „das, was den Mitgliedern einer wissenschaftlichen Gemeinschaft gemeinsam ist". Eine wissenschaftliche Gemeinschaft besteht folgerichtig „aus Menschen, die ein Paradigma teilen". Kuhn führt aus, dass „von einem Paradigma angenommen wird, dass es die meisten Beobachtungen und Experimente, welche für die Fachleute jener Wissenschaft leicht zugänglich sind, erfolgreich erklärt". Warnend führt der weltweit zitierte Autor aus, dass ein Paradigma zu einer immensen Einschränkung des Gesichtskreises führt und zu einem beträchtlichen Widerstand gegen einen Paradigmenwechsel (vgl. Kuhn, 1996).

Damit sind wir schließlich bei der Zahnmedizin angekommen, und zwar auf dem Wege über die ethische Definition ärztlichen Handelns durch Hippokrates und über die Einführung des durch Galilei begründeten und von Claude Bernard in die Medizin eingeführten, auf wissenschaftlicher Beobachtung und Experiment beruhenden Reduktionismus. Die Zahnmedizin ist keine sehr alte Disziplin der Medizin. Aktivitäten zur Professionalisierung der Zahnheilkunde sowie die ersten vorsichtigen Versuche, zahnheilkundliche Tätigkeit auf wissenschaftlicher Erkenntnis aufzubauen, begannen, als die Medizin insgesamt anfing, sich naturwissenschaftlich zu orientieren. Diese Phase der methodischen Neuorientierung ist in der Medizin gut 150 Jahre alt, hat im „restaurativen" Fach der Zahnheilkunde aber noch keine lange Tradition. Es ist vielmehr in aller Nüchternheit festzustellen, dass das Paradigma „Handwerkermodell", das möglicherweise bei der Bewältigung der Probleme in der Vergangenheit geholfen hat, für die Gegenwart und die Zukunft nicht mehr ausreicht. Dieses Modell konnte anfangs den Anforderungen eines zahnärztlichen Unterrichts genügen. Wissenschaftlich kreativ war es nie, worauf möglicherweise die nicht zu verleugnende Lethargie in der zahnärztlichen Wissenschaft zurückzuführen ist. Dem Praktiker konnte es keine Hilfestellung geben, da es die Komplexität und Kompliziertheit der Zahnheilkunde negierte. Für die Formulierung einer zukunftsweisenden Qualitätssicherung, die ja Innovation und nicht Starre auslösen sollte, war es vollkommen untauglich. Und auch für die Herausforderung, eine evidenzbasierte Zahnheilkunde zu begründen, wird es vollkommen untauglich sein.

„Evidence-based Dentistry" ist kein Kinderspiel, das man nebenbei ohne tiefsinnige Gedanken gewinnen kann. Die Zeit, in der Wissenschaft und Praxis ihre Tätigkeit auf der Grundlage der einfachen Gedankengänge des Handwerkermodells aufgebaut und begründet haben, ist endgültig vorüber und es heißt deshalb, davon Abschied zu nehmen. Aller Abschied ist schwer, insbesondere der Abschied von lieb gewonnenen und einfachen Gedanken. Abschied bedeutet Unsicherheit verbreitende Unruhe, aber auch Herausforderung. Die Herausforderung nämlich, die Unsicherheit in eine motivierende und dadurch produktive Unruhe umzuändern. Auch das ist nicht leicht. Ganz im Gegenteil, es erfordert harte Arbeit.

1 Dentistry as a scientific discipline

Michael Heners, Karlsruhe

1.1 Preliminary note

Dentistry, like medicine as a whole, is increasingly being challenged by issues that compel it to clarify the foundations of its activity. One of these issues is the basis of scientific evidence that underlies dental decision-making. This in turn implies questions regarding dentistry as a scientific discipline.

The need for dentistry to be scientifically based has been recognized by the legislator and enshrined in law in Germany. The Law on the Exercise of the Dental Profession provides as follows: "Dentistry is the professional identification and treatment, based on dental scientific knowledge, of diseases of the teeth, mouth and jaw. A disease shall be deemed to be any abnormal manifestation in the mouth and jaw, including tooth malalignment and missing teeth" (cf. Gesetze für Ärzte und andere Heilberufe, 1995).

By this law, the legislator not only defined the dentist's field of activity – "identification and treatment of diseases of the teeth, mouth and jaw" – but also stipulated unequivocally that this activity must be conducted professionally and be based on scientific knowledge. What then is the meaning of "scientific knowledge"?

Scientific knowledge is often equated with statements that result from the formal working of scientific institutions and derive their authority from the attributes of these institutions – e.g. a university or academy, the status of a professor, Ph.D., M.A., etc. Universities and other institutions of higher learning were in fact established to provide science with a space to unfold, whether it be on the level of research or teaching or both. However, the very fact that all such idealistically founded spaces also require a formal apparatus in order to function gives rise to potential discrepancies between the initial ideal and the formal apparatus, between the idealistic aspiration and the formal reality, resulting in a displacement of the original task. Such trends result not only in rigidity but also in a new orientation, which no doubt always has the same objective, namely that of bringing a science that has succumbed to formalistic complacency back to its original task or primordial intention. The novel scientific approach known as "evidence-based medicine" is an example of this phenomenon.

1.2 Task of dental science

What is the task, or primordial intention, of dental science? According to the German Dentistry Law, the answer must be: to describe and make verifiable the identification and treatment of diseases of the teeth, mouth and jaw in all their complexity and actual complication. Since dentistry is a purpose-directed science, this description is not undertaken for its own sake but is intended to enable the dentist to come to the aid of the person seeking help and to do so by means of verifiable methods. As both a theoretical and a practical science, dentistry – like medicine as a whole – lacks an appropriate orientation unless it has an ethical basis.

Finally, the descriptions of diseases of the teeth, mouth and jaw must be verifiable. This means that the methods used for observing and describing the complex and diverse dental reality must conform to logical and unambiguously defined rules. This is what is known as the scientific methodology (cf. Heners, 1985). Since the relevant methodology is usually highly complicated and requires specific expertise, the knowledge accruing from its application must be acquired through specific study. It is therefore appropriate and indeed essential for the exercise of dentistry to be conditional on study and for the practice of scientific activity to be bound up with the institutions that underpin the working methods. This is at any rate the case if dentistry is to be scientifically based and practised, as is nowadays considered desirable.

Therapeutic measures are always "interventions". On this point, Schipperges (1970) writes: "The specific activity of the doctor consists in the fact that he must intervene when asked for help in order to avert affliction. The resulting intervention always affects the integrity of a human being, for the doctor intervenes not only with his knife but also with drugs and, indeed, with his advice and, as the case may be, with his perplexity as well." In view of the uncertainty of medical action, it is understandable that the practice of scientifically based medicine must be preceded by a determination of the applicable ethical context (see Fig. 1-1).

The principles of "nihil nocere" (cause no harm or hurt) and "solus aegroti salus" (act for the benefit of the patient only) laid down in the Hippocratic Oath impose limits on medical activity to this day (cf. Ankermann, 1991).

1.3 The Galilean epistemological principle and reductionistic thinking

The discovery of the methodological approach of the modern natural sciences – rejection of authority in matters of scientific knowledge and the basing of general principles solely on observation and experiment (Galileo Galilei's "method of inductive reasoning", see Fig. 1-2) – is relevant to the scientific

1.3 The Galilean epistemological principle and reductionistic thinking

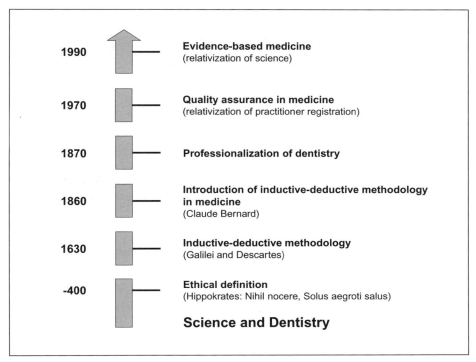

Figure 1-1: Stages in the evolution of the scientific status of medicine and dentistry

status of dentistry in that, centuries after its discovery, Claude Bernard in 1860 introduced this methodology into medicine for describing the regular laws of the healthy and diseased body. The methodology remains more or less binding to this day in the "classical medicine" of every country in the world.

However, the consistent and/or rigorous application of the Galilean epistemological principle has not only led to an enormous and incredible expansion of medical knowledge and the art of medicine, but also rendered the field of medical knowledge so vast that an overall view has become impossible. In the end this methodology proved feasible only if one was prepared to sacrifice the "desire to see the whole picture". This notion was formulated by René Descartes in the following terms some 350 years ago: "If a problem is so complex that you cannot solve it all at once, divide it into a number of sub-problems each small enough for you to be able to solve them separately." Modern medicine has learned to apply this "principle of reduction" to the diagnosis and healing of diseases which could previously be neither diagnosed nor healed. However, medicine thereby tacitly accepted an approach whereby both sick and healthy people were seen "solely in reductionistic terms" (cf. Zenner, 2000; Heners, 1977).

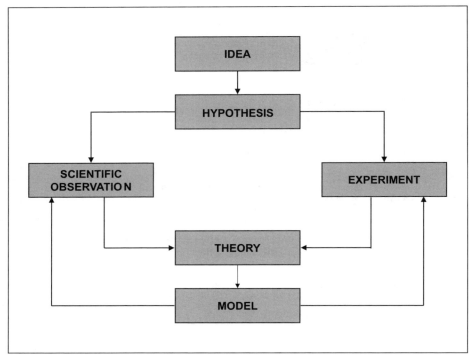

Figure 1-2: Epistemological principle of induction and deduction

1.4 Discrepancy between medical activity and scientific abstraction

The plethora of information resulting from this methodology has in our time inevitably called into question two parameters hitherto regarded as unshakeable foundations of the professional practice of medicine: the claim to absoluteness of both the registration of medical practitioners and scientific information. After all, since medical activity can be appropriate and successful only if it takes account of the patient "as a whole", the question was bound to arise whether the available information could be assembled by the practitioner into a logical unity on the spot – i. e. in the treatment of an individual patient. The demand for "quality assurance in medicine" thus appears as an attempt to restore the complication of medical activity to the practitioner's consciousness. If medical activity that lacks an accompanying basis of quality assurance is called into question, registration of practitioners becomes a more relative criterion.

The formulation of the notions of an evidence-based medicine goes further. It calls into question scientific information itself, as well as the medical decisions based on it. This approach is directed towards both medical science

1.4 Discrepancy between medical activity and scientific abstraction

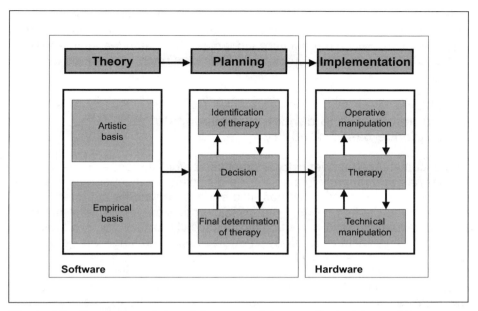

Figure 1-3: Parameters of dental therapy and therapeutic decision-making

and the practitioner, who, after all, is required to solve clinical problems. The application of a scientific methodology must become compulsory if relevant and undistorted information is to be available as a basis for practical decision-making. The practitioner should look more closely at the methodology he deploys in relation to his own problems, while applying the best available knowledge.

"Science" and "medical activity" are thus found to be a pair of concepts that have proved their worth in the last hundred years, but whose efficiency has reached its limits, so that corrections, which will hopefully be successful, have become necessary. The idea of basing medical activity solely on "scientific" criteria has after all met with healthy scepticism from the beginning. As Sir William Osler, the Canadian-born British specialist in internal diseases, wrote at the beginning of the twentieth century: "The practice of medicine is an art based on science." This formulation was intended to draw attention to the discrepancy between medical activity and scientific abstraction. The determining parameters of dental activity are summarized in Figure 1-3 (see Fig. 1-3).

The software of dental action (what is not visible to the eye) is distinguished from its hardware, i.e. classical manipulative activity. Schipperges (see above) defined medical activity as an intervention affecting the integrity of the human subject not only with the knife and drugs but also with the doctor's advice and his perplexity; in addition to this, however, the specific practice of the dentist includes the application of his restorative art. Furthermore, the dentist's intervention is not effected invisibly, but is exposed to the patient's observing eye. Hence the dentist's judgement that precedes an intervention and accompanies it to its completion will be confirmed – or not, as the case may be.

1.5 Paradigm shift in dentistry: challenges of an evidence-based dentistry

The circumstance that dentistry is practised before the observing eye of the patient has permanently influenced the discipline's conception of itself. It is a conception of dentistry that has also been described as the "craft model" (cf. Heners & Walther, 2000). The classical decision-making parameters of this model, which have been applied uncritically to this day, are banalities such as: "If everything is always done properly, nothing can go wrong", or "Beautiful is better", or "The better is the enemy of the good", and – what might be described as the encapsulation of all economic considerations – "Dearer is healthier!" The diabolical thing about these banalities – as with most of their kind – is that they seem so plausible as to need no further proof. Yet they are false! Even so, these banalities substantially determine the debate among specialists in dentistry. They are so to speak the scientific paradigm, from which – because they are beautifully banal and simple – one does not wish to part.

The historian of science Thomas S. Kuhn defines a "paradigm" as that what the members of a scientific community share. It follows that a scientific community consists of men who share a paradigm. According to Kuhn, a paradigm is expected successfully to explain most of the observations and experiments that are readily accessible to specialists in a given science. This world-renowned author warns that a paradigm gives rise to an immense restriction of one's field of view and that a paradigm shift generates appreciable resistance (cf. Kuhn, 1996).

This finally brings us to dentistry – by way of Hippocrates's ethical definition of medical activity and the introduction of reductionism based on scientific observation and experiment, due to Galilei and introduced to medicine by Claude Bernard. Dentistry is not a very old medical discipline. The professionalization of dentistry and the first cautious attempts to place dental activity on a foundation of scientific knowledge commenced when medicine as a whole began to adopt a natural-science orientation. This phase of methodological reorientation is over 150 years old in medicine, but does not yet have a long tradition in the dental "restorative" discipline. It has to be soberly recognized that the "craft model" paradigm, although it may have helped to solve problems in the past, no longer suffices for the present and the future. At first this model met the requirements of dental education adequately. The fact that it was never scientifically creative may explain the undeniable lethargy that exists in dental science. It could not help the practitioner because it disregarded the complexity and complication of dentistry. It was totally unfit to formulate a future-oriented form of quality assurance, which, after all, was supposed to stimulate innovation and not rigidity. Nor will it be in any way fit to meet the challenge of establishing an evidence-based dentistry.

"Evidence-based dentistry" is not a children's game that can be won just like that without exercising minds unduly. The days when science and practice could build and base their activity on the foundation of the simple notions of the craft model are gone once and for all. The model is too banal and must therefore be given a final farewell. Parting is always difficult, especially where fondly nurtured, simple ideas are concerned. Parting entails not only a state of unease that spreads uncertainty, but also a challenge. The challenge is to convert the uncertainty into an unease that is motivating and hence productive. That too is not easy. On the contrary, it calls for hard work.

1.6 Literatur/References

Ankermann, E.: Behandlungsstandard und -spielraum in der Zahnmedizin aus haftungsrechtlicher Sicht. Dtsch Zahnärztl Z 46 (1991), 253–256

Gesetze für Ärzte und andere Heilberufe. München 1995

Heners, M.: Erkenntnistheoretische Modelle in der Zahn-, Mund- und Kieferheilkunde. Dtsch Zahnärztl Z 32 (1977), 841–847

Heners, M.: Methodik als Prinzip der Wissenschaft. Quintessenz 43 (1985), 47–50

Heners, M., Walther, W.: Zahnärztliche Qualitätssicherung. Schweiz Monatsschr Zahnmed, 110 (2000), 51–57

Kuhn, T. S.: The Structure of Scientific Revolutions. Chicago 1996

Schipperges, H.: Moderne Medizin im Spiegel der Geschichte. Stuttgart 1970

Zenner, H. P.: Die Physik und Grundfragen ärztlichen Handelns. Dtsch Ärztebl 97 (2000), A-164, Heft 4

2 Entscheidungsfindung auf der Grundlage der besten externen wissenschaftlichen Evidenz: Eine Herausforderung für den Wissenschaftler und den Praktiker

Derek Richards, Oxford

2.1 Einleitung

Tagtäglich treffen Zahnärzte eine Vielzahl von Entscheidungen über die bestmögliche Behandlung ihrer Patienten. Bei diesem Entscheidungsprozess spielen viele unterschiedliche Einflussfaktoren eine Rolle (vgl. Abb. 2-1).

Die wissenschaftliche Evidenz ist nur einer dieser Einflussfaktoren, allerdings ein wichtiger. Mit der Entwicklung evidenz-basierter Gesundheitsver-

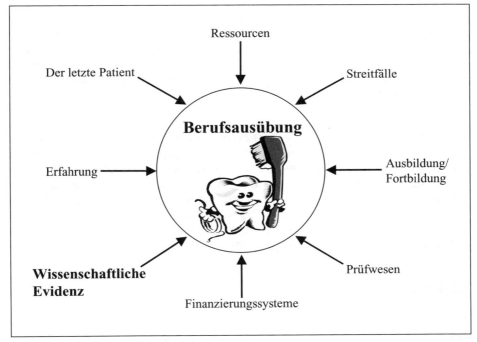

Abbildung 2-1: Faktoren, die die Behandlungsentscheidung beeinflussen

sorgung, die wie folgt definiert wurde (vgl. Sackett et al., 1996), hat sie zunehmend an Bedeutung gewonnen:

„Evidenz-basierte Medizin (EBM) ist der gewissenhafte, ausdrückliche und vernünftige Gebrauch der gegenwärtig besten externen wissenschaftlichen Evidenz für Entscheidungen über die medizinische Versorgung individueller Patienten."

David Sackett

Es handelt sich hierbei um einen Problemlösungsansatz, bei dem man die klinische Beurteilung und die bestmögliche zur Verfügung stehende Evidenz nutzt, um die bestmögliche Versorgung für den betreffenden Patienten sicherzustellen.

2.2 Warum sind Veränderungen erforderlich?

Alle Gesundheitssysteme stehen unter einem gewissen Druck, und es gibt vier wesentliche externe auslösende Faktoren dafür:

- höhere Lebenserwartung,
- neue Technologien/Materialien,
- Wandel des Krankheitspanoramas,
- steigendes Verbraucherbewusstsein.

Die meisten Industrieländer verzeichnen einen zunehmenden Anteil älterer Menschen an der Bevölkerung, und diese Gruppe verursacht – zusammen mit den ganz Jungen – den größten Anteil an den Gesundheitsausgaben. Für die Zahnheilkunde bedeutet dies älter werdende Patienten mit umfangreichen restaurativen Versorgungen, die künftig über viele Jahre kostenintensive Maßnahmen zu deren Erhaltung bzw. Wiederherstellung in Anspruch nehmen werden.

Es werden kontinuierlich neue Technologien entwickelt, z. B. zahnärztliche Implantate, Laserbehandlungen, Gore-Tex für parodontales Reattachment und vieles andere. Das Kariesaufkommen hat sich verändert, jüngere Patienten haben immer weniger Karies. Darüber hinaus haben wir es in zunehmendem Maße mit besser informierten Patienten zu tun, die mehr Mitsprache in Bezug auf ihre gesundheitliche Versorgung haben möchten bzw. einfordern. Dieses gestiegene Gesundheitsbewusstsein ist ein Symptom des steigenden Verbraucherbewusstseins.

2.3 Probleme bei der Umsetzung von Innovationen

Wenn neue Erkenntnisse oder neue Technologien vorliegen, würden diese im Idealfall in das Gesundheitssystem übernommen. In der Realität gibt es hier aber – wie in Abb. 2-2 dargestellt – zwei wesentliche Probleme: Der

2.3 Probleme bei der Umsetzung von Innovationen

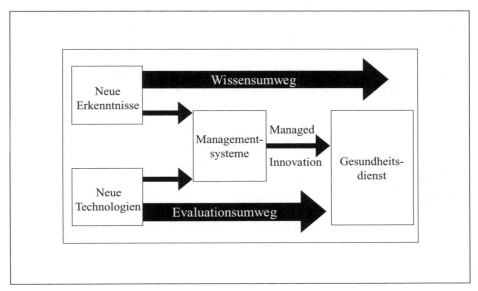

Abbildung 2-2: Innovationsumweg

Wissens„umweg", wenn entweder neue Erkenntnisse nicht vorliegen oder diese erst nach vielen Jahren, wenn der Nachweis für ihre Wirksamkeit schon lange erbracht wurde, in die allgemeine Gesundheitsversorgung Eingang finden, so z. B. bei Thrombolytika oder Fissurenversieglern. Und auf der anderen Seite das Problem, wenn neue Verfahren sehr schnell von den im Gesundheitswesen Verantwortlichen aufgegriffen werden, obwohl der effizienteste Wirkungsbereich noch gar nicht sorgfältig dokumentiert ist. Orthopantomogramme (OPGs) sind hierfür ein Beispiel; sie sind in der Oralchirurgie, oralen Pathologie und in der kieferorthopädischen Diagnose sehr nutzbringend, jedoch in der Karies- oder Parodontaldiagnose, wozu sie von vielen Zahnärzten eingesetzt werden, nur von sehr begrenztem Nutzen.

Es gibt auch eine Reihe interner Beweggründe für eine evidenz-basierte Gesundheitsversorgung, die für alle Heilberufe gelten:

- Es werden neue wissenschaftlich gesicherte Erkenntnisse (Evidenz) vorgelegt, die die Patientenversorgung verbessern können.
- Hiervon erhalten wir nicht automatisch Kenntnis.
- Wissensstand und Leistungserbringung verschlechtern sich im Lauf der Zeit.
- Durch traditionelle Fortbildung wird die Leistungserbringung nicht verbessert.
- Es ist belegt, dass der evidenz-basierte Ansatz Ärzte und Zahnärzte auf einem aktuellen Stand hält.

Bei 500 oder mehr zahnärztlichen und 30.000 biomedizinischen Zeitschriften, die jährlich veröffentlicht werden, kann es natürlich leicht passieren, dass man Informationen über neue Erkenntnisse übersieht. Es ist auch nicht sichergestellt, dass man neue Informationen dann erhält, wenn sie wichtig sind, obwohl in einigen Ländern für die Verbreitung wissenschaftlicher Evidenz, die als wichtig erachtet wird, Sorge getragen wird. So werden z. B. im Vereinigten Königreich „Effectiveness Bulletins" veröffentlicht und an die relevanten Berufsvertreter weitergeleitet; es kann aber immer noch passieren, dass sie nicht gelesen werden.

Obwohl mancher es nur schwer akzeptieren kann, werden viele zustimmen, dass sich unser Wissensstand und unsere Leistung im Lauf der Zeit verschlechtern.

„Die Hälfte dessen, was man Sie als Medizinstudent lehrt, wird sich in zehn Jahren als falsch herausgestellt haben. Das Problem ist, dass keiner Ihrer Lehrer weiß, welche Hälfte das ist."
C. Sidney Burwell (1893–1956)

Die traditionelle Fortbildung ändert nur selten Verhaltensweisen. Es hat sich allerdings gezeigt, dass der evidenz-basierte Ansatz zu deutlichen Verhaltensänderungen führt. In einer von Shin durchgeführten Studie wurde die Leistungserbringung von Absolventen der McMaster Medical School, die einen evidenz-basierten Ansatz in der Lehre zu Grunde legt, mit der von Absolventen einer traditionellen medizinischen Hochschule verglichen. Ein Vergleich der Behandlung bei Bluthochdruck 10 Jahre nach Examensabschluss ergab, dass die McMaster-Absolventen neuere Behandlungsmethoden anwendeten als ihre Kollegen von der traditionellen medizinischen Hochschule (vgl. Shin, Haynes und Johnston, 1993).

2.4 Evidenzgrade

Wissenschaftliche Evidenz steht in unterschiedlicher Form zur Verfügung. Wie soll also die Klassifikation erfolgen? Als Ausgangspunkt sinnvoll ist die bekannte Einteilung der Agency for Health Care Policy and Research (vgl. AHCPR, 1992):

– höchste Evidenz aus mindestens einem veröffentlichten systematischen Review über eine multiple, methodisch hochwertige randomisierte kontrollierte Studie,
– höchste Evidenz aus mindestens einer veröffentlichten methodisch hochwertigen, randomisierten kontrollierten Studie mit adäquater Stichprobengröße und unter adäquaten klinischen Untersuchungsbedingungen,
– Evidenz aus methodisch hochwertigen experimentellen Studien aus mehr als einem Zentrum oder von mehr als einer Forschungsgruppe,
– Evidenz aus methodisch hochwertigen randomisierten Studien, einzelnen

Vorher-Nachher-Studien, Kohortenstudien, Fallserien oder Fall-Kontroll-Studien,
– Expertenmeinungen auf der Basis klinischer Evidenz, deskriptiver Studien oder Berichte klinischer Konsensuskomitees.

Diese Einteilung bezieht sich jedoch nur auf therapeutische Fragestellungen. Wichtig ist es zu bedenken, dass die wissenschaftliche Evidenz der zu Grunde liegenden Fragestellung gerecht werden muss. Für prognostische Fragestellungen sind eher Kohortenstudien geeignet. Wenn wir eine Forschungsfrage untersuchen möchten, muss das bestgeeignete Studiendesign zur Beantwortung der Fragestellung zu Grunde gelegt werden (vgl. Tab. 2-1).

Tabelle 2-1: Adäquanz von Studiendesigns

	Qualitativ	Querschnitt	Fallkontrolliert	Kohorten-Studie	RCT	Systematischer Review
Diagnose				☆	☆☆	☆☆☆
Therapie				☆	☆☆	☆☆☆
Prognose				☆☆☆		
Screening			☆	☆	☆☆	☆☆☆
Ansichten/ Einschätzungen/ Wahrnehmungen	☆☆☆					
Management-Innovation	☆		☆	☆	☆☆	☆☆☆
Hypothesengenerierung	☆☆☆					
Prävalenz		☆☆☆				

☆ Die Anzahl der Sternchen weist das am besten geeignete Studiendesign aus

2.5 Evidenz-Basis in der Zahnheilkunde

Wie ist die vorliegende wissenschaftliche Evidenz quantitativ einzuordnen? Dr. R. Niederman, Harvard, hat die Anzahl randomisierter kontrollierter Studien für verschiedene Fachbereiche in der Medizin mit denen für die Zahnheilkunde verglichen (vgl. Niederman, 1999). Die Zahnheilkunde ist hier mit randominiserten kontrollierten Studien zahlenmäßig nur sehr schwach vertreten. Innerhalb der zahnärztlichen Fachgebiete wurden von den Parodontologen die meisten randomisierten klinischen Studien durchgeführt, von den Endodontologen die wenigsten.

Eine in Wales durchgeführte Studie über die Evidenz-Basis in Bezug auf Studien über orale Erkrankungen (vgl. Health Evidence Bulletins Wales, 1998) zeigt, dass ein großer Teil dieser Studien den niedrigen Evidenzgraden zuzuordnen ist (vgl. Tabelle 2-2).

Tabelle 2-2: Evidenz-Basis in der Zahnheilkunde						
	Anzahl Statements	Grad der wissenschaftlichen Evidenz[1]				
		I[2]	II	III	IV	V
Karies	26	9 (7)	0	8	4	17
Parodonto-pathien	14	13 (8)	0	1	1	2
Dento-faziale Anomalien	15	1	0	0	1	6
Mundkrebs	10	0	0	0	11	7
Kiefergelenk-Erkrankungen	7	0	0	1	0	6
Abrasion	12	0	0	0	10	4
Verletzungen der Zähne	16	0	1	3	5	9
Angeborene Anomalien	7	0	0	0	1	7
Insgesamt	**107**	**23 (15)**	**1**	**13**	**33**	**58**

[1] Evidenzgrade gemäß der AHCPR-Einteilung, Grad I hat die höchste Entscheidungssicherheit, Grad V die geringste.
[2] Die Zahlen in Klammern unter Grad I beziehen sich auf die aktuelle Anzahl systematischer Reviews; die höhere wird genannt, da einige Reviews mehr als ein Statement beantworten.

Quelle: Health Evidence Bulletins Wales, 1998

Die derzeitige Basis wissenschaftlicher Evidenz in der Zahnheilkunde kann also gemäß dem Tortendiagramm in Abbildung 2-3 (vgl. Abb. 2-3) dargestellt werden. Das Ziel ist es, sich auf einen Punkt hinzubewegen, wo wir entweder von allen Maßnahmen, die wir erbringen, wissen, dass sie „mehr nutzen als schaden" oder Inhalt einer gut angelegten Studie sind (vgl. Abb. 2-4).

„Die Tatsache, dass eine Meinung weitverbreitet ist, ist keinerlei Beweis dafür, dass sie nicht vollkommen absurd ist; angesichts der Dummheit der Mehrheit der Menschen ist die Wahrscheinlichkeit, dass eine weitverbreitete Ansicht töricht ist, höher als dass sie vernünftig ist."

Bertrand Russell (1872–1970), „Marriage and Morals" (1929), Kap. 5

2.5 Evidenz-Basis in der Zahnheilkunde

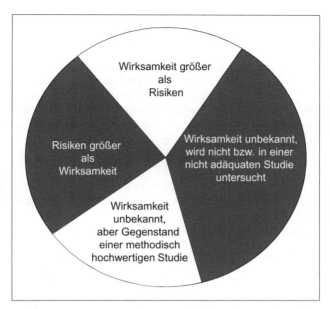

Abbildung 2-3: Einschätzung der aktuellen Evidenz-Basis für zahnärztliche Maßnahmen

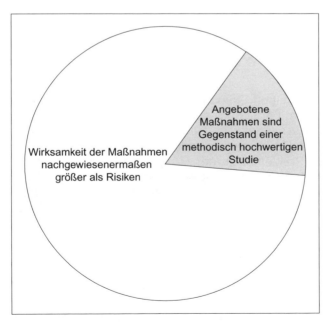

Abbildung 2-4: Angestrebte Zielsetzung für die Evidenz-Basis zahnärztlicher Maßnahmen

2.6 Forschung und Anwendung in der evidenz-basierten Zahnheilkunde

Obwohl die Kapitelüberschrift im Hinblick auf den Wissenschaftler und den Praktiker unterscheidet, sollte der gesamte Berufsstand einen „wissenschaftlichen Zugang" haben. Man kann allerdings den Berufsstand in die folgenden beiden Gruppen einteilen: Die ANWENDER der Evidenz – und dies sollte der gesamte Berufsstand sein – und die in der Forschung Tätigen oder die MACHER.

Die „Anwender" müssen:
– eine Fragestellung oder verschiedene Fragestellungen in Bezug auf den gegenwärtigen gesundheitlichen Zustand eines Patienten adäquat formulieren können,
– wissen, welche Quellen der Evidenz eingesetzt werden sollten und wie man Zugang dazu erhält,
– in der Lage sein, die gefundene Evidenz kritisch zu bewerten,
– Kritik üben, wenn Informationen in der wissenschaftlichen Literatur mangelhaft dargestellt/erläutert werden.

Dunn et al. (1997) fanden heraus, dass 75% der Krankenschwestern Statistiken nicht verstehen und 70% nicht in der Lage sind, eine Forschungsarbeit kritisch zu bewerten. Vine und Hastings (1994) stellten fest, dass die meisten Ärzte mit Ja antworten, wenn sie gefragt werden, ob sie täglich eine Tablette einnehmen würden, wenn sie damit das Risiko, an einem Herzanfall zu sterben, um 50% reduzieren könnten. Wird jedoch als Frage formuliert, ob sie dies über 10–20 Jahre tun würden, wenn ihr Risiko damit von 2/1000 auf 1/1000 verringert würde, hält sich die Begeisterung sehr in Grenzen!

Die „Macher" betreiben Grundlagenforschung; dies ist von essentieller Bedeutung für den Fortschritt der Zahnheilkunde und für die Sekundärforschung oder systematische Reviews, die immer mehr an Bedeutung gewinnen. Sackett (1979) stellt allerdings in seiner Untersuchung ein breites Spektrum von Problemen in der Grundlagenforschung fest (vgl. Tab. 2-3). Schor und Karten (1966) dokumentieren in besorgniserregendem Umfang statistische Probleme in Beiträgen, die im Journal der American Medical Association veröffentlicht wurden. Nach Altman (1991) hatte sich dieser Sachstand einige Jahre später kaum verbessert.

Mulrow (1987) analysierte 50 Reviews, die im Zeitraum 1985–1986 in vier größeren Zeitschriften erschienen. Er stellte fest, dass 49 keine Angaben zur Methodik enthielten und 47 nur unzureichende Zusammenfassungen. Er zog daraus die Schlussfolgerung: „Für medizinische Reviews finden derzeit noch nicht routinemäßig wissenschaftliche Verfahren zur Identifikation, Bewertung und Zusammenfassung der Information Anwendung."

Tabelle 2-3: Fehler im Studiendesign

	Prozentsatz von Arbeiten, die Probleme aufwarfen
	%
Planung	5
Design	22
Ausführung	18
Datenverarbeitung	5
Interpretation	6

1993 analysierte Silagy Reviews in Zeitschriften zur Primärversorgung (vgl. Silagy, 1993). Obwohl eine Verbesserung konstatiert werden konnte, gibt es hier noch sehr viel zu tun. Es ist anzunehmen, dass wir uns in der Zahnheilkunde bestenfalls auf dem Stand befinden, den Mulrow 1987 für die Medizin konstatierte; möglicherweise aber noch auf einem schlechteren Niveau.

2.7 Welche Herausforderungen stehen für die Zukunft an?

Entsprechend muss der zahnärztliche Berufsstand:
- in der Lage sein, die richtigen Fragen zu stellen,
- wissen, wo man Evidenz sucht,
- kritisch urteilen können,
- Kritik aufzeigen.

Anforderungen an die Primärforscher:
- eine bessere Ausbildung für die Forschung,
- Schärfung des Bewusstseins für das adäquate Forschungsdesign,
- optimierte Präsentation und Verbreitung der Ergebnisse.

Anforderungen an die Sekundärforscher:
- eine bessere Ausbildung im Hinblick auf die Methodologie für systematische Reviews,
- mehr systematische Reviews,
- Verbesserung der Verbreitung.

2.8 Die Verbreitung evidenz-basierter Erkenntnisse und Implementationsstrategien

Die Verbreitung evidenz-basierter Erkenntnisse stellt ein Problem dar. Zwei aktuelle Beispiele aus Großbritannien verdeutlichen dies. Es wurden zwei umfassende Reviews zur Fragestellung der Förderung der Mundgesundheit durchgeführt (vgl. Sprod, Anderson und Treasure, 1966; Kay und Locker, 1998); dennoch war die Mehrheit der Zahnärzte bei Nachfrage darüber nicht informiert. Noch weniger Aufmerksamkeit fanden evidenz-basierte Leitlinien über den Einsatz von Röntgenaufnahmen in der zahnärztlichen Literatur, obwohl diese von der Faculty of General Dental Practitioners (1999) erarbeitet wurden.

Dies leitet über zur Implementierung. Hier steht man wahrscheinlich vor den größten Herausforderungen, obwohl auf diesem Gebiet viel geforscht wurde und die Maßnahmen, die die größte Übereinstimmung in Bezug auf ihre Effizienz zeigen, in einer Reihe von Cochrane-Reviews identifiziert wurden (vgl. Bero et al., 1998). Die höchste Effizienz haben danach:

- Praxisvisite,
- Erinnerungssysteme,
- interaktive Fortbildung,
- mehrgleisige Implementationsstrategie.

Die geringste Effizienz haben:
- Informationsmaterial,
- traditionelle Fortbildungsveranstaltung.

2.9 Ausblick

Zusammenfassend kann man sagen, dass die beste Gesundheitsversorgung diejenige ist, die auf der besten, verfügbaren Evidenz basiert und bei der alle Maßnahmen, deren Wirksamkeit nicht nachgewiesen ist, ausgeschaltet werden. D. h. also, dass die Maßnahmen, die ergriffen werden, von der höchstmöglichen Effizienz für diejenigen Patientengruppen sind, die aller Wahrscheinlichkeit nach davon profitieren, und die Maßnahmen die höchstmögliche Qualität haben.

Ein evidenz-basierter Ansatz in der Zahnheilkunde kann dazu beitragen, dieses Ziel zu erreichen. Ein solcher Ansatz kann unter den folgenden fünf Schwerpunkten zusammengefasst werden:

- Entscheidungen sollten auf der Grundlage der besten, verfügbaren Evidenz getroffen werden.
- Basis ist das klinische Problem des Patienten.
- Es gilt, die wissenschaftliche Evidenz aller verfügbarer Quellen einzubeziehen.
- Die Schlussfolgerungen aufgrund der kritisch bewerteten Evidenz müssen klinisch relevant sein.
- Die Mitglieder des Berufsstandes müssen ihren Leistungsstandard regelmäßig überprüfen.

2.9 Ausblick

Dies ist nicht neu und die meisten guten Zahnärzte haben ihren Beruf auch bislang nach diesen Kriterien ausgeübt. Dies belegt abschließend ein Zitat, das die Annäherung an die Fragestellungen, die evidenz-basierte Verfahren an die Zahnheilkunde herantragen, zusammenfasst und nahezu 400 Jahren alt ist:

„Steht am Anfang Gewissheit, so wird der Mensch bei Zweifeln enden; gibt er sich aber damit zufrieden, dass am Anfang Zweifel stehen, so wird er am Ende Gewissheit erlangen."
Francis Bacon (1561–1626), „The Advancement of Learning" (1605)

2 Use of best evidence in making decisions: a challenge for the scientist and practitioner

Derek Richards, Oxford

2.1 Introduction

Everyday dentists make many decisions about how best to treat their patients. The influences on this decision making process are many and varied (see Fig. 2-1).

Evidence is only one of these influences, but an important one. The role of evidence had become increasingly important with the development of evi-

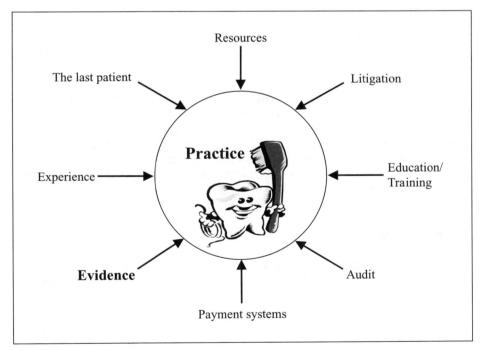

Figure 2-1: Influences on decisions

dence-based health care, which has been defined (cf. Sackett et al., 1996) as:

"Evidence-based medicine is the conscientious, explicit, and judicious use of current best evidence in making decisions about the care of individual patients."

David Sackett

This is a problem solving approach using clinical judgement and the best available evidence to ensure the most appropriate care for a particular patient.

2.2 Drivers for change

All health care systems are under pressure and there are four fundamental external driving forces for this:

– ageing population,
– new technology/materials,
– changing patterns of disease,
– consumerism.

Most developing countries have an ageing population and this group together with the very young consumes the greatest amount of health care spending. In dentistry we have an ageing cohort of patients with heavily restored mouths which will require expensive repair and maintenance for many years to come.

New technology is constantly emerging e.g. dental implants, laser treatments, Gore-Tex for periodontal reattachment and many more. The pattern of caries has changed with a younger cohort of patients with low caries levels now emerging. Increasingly we are seeing more informed (knowledgeable) patients who want and demand a greater say in their health care. This increased awareness is a symptom of a more widespread phenomenon of consumerism.

2.3 Innovation bypass

In an ideal situation when new knowledge or new technology emerge it would be filtered into the health system. However in reality there are two main bypasses to this (see Fig. 2-2):

– the Knowledge bypass when new knowledge is either missed or not brought into mainstream health care until many years after its effectiveness is already well established e.g. Thrombolytic drugs or fissure sealants,

2.3 Innovation bypass

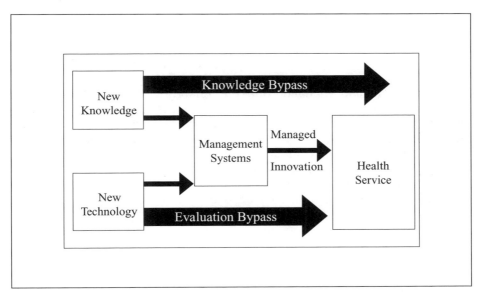

Figure 2-2: Innovation bypass

– and those where new technology is rapidly taken up by health care professionals even though its most effective use has not been properly evaluated, e.g. OPGs which although useful for oral surgery, oral pathology and orthodontic diagnosis have very limited use for caries and periodontal diagnosis for which they are used by many practitioners.

There are also a number of internal drivers for evidence-based health care, which are common to all professions.

– New evidence is being found which can improve patient care.
– We do not automatically receive new evidence.
– Knowledge and performance deteriorate with time.
– Traditional continuing education does not improve performance.
– The evidence-based approach has been shown to keep practitioners up to date.

With 500 or more dental journals and 30000 biomedical journals published annually it is easy to miss new information. It is also unusual to receive new information when it is important although some countries do disseminate evidence they consider important. For example in the UK effectiveness bulletins are published and distributed to relevant professionals, however they may still not be read.

Although unpalatable to some, many will agree our knowledge levels and performance does deteriorate with the passage of time.

"Half of what you are taught as medical students will in ten years have been shown to be wrong, and the trouble is none of your teachers know which half."

C. Sidney Burwell (1893–1956)

Traditional continuing education does not change behaviour. However, the evidence based approach has been shown to change behaviour. A study conducted by Shin compared the performance of medical graduates from McMaster Medical school, which uses an evidence-based approach to its teaching with a traditional medical school (cf. Shin, Haynes and Johnston, 1993). Looking at their treatment of hypertension 10 years following graduation they found that McMaster graduates where using more up to date treatment methods than their colleagues from the traditional medical school.

2.4 Levels of evidence

Evidence comes in many forms, so how do we grade it. A useful starting point is this well known grading from the Agency for Health Care Policy and Research (cf. AHCPR, 1992):

- strong evidence from at least one published systematic review of multiple well designed randomised controlled trial,
- strong evidence from at least one published properly designed randomised controlled trial of appropriate size and in an appropriate clinical setting,
- evidence from well designed experimental studies from more than one centre or research group,
- evidence from published well designed trials without randomisation, single pre-post cohort time, series or matched case controlled studies,
- opinions of respected authorities, based on clinical evidence, descriptive studies or reports of clinical consensus committees.

However this only refers to therapy. What is important to remember is that the evidence must be appropriate for the question asked. Therefore if we are concerned with prognosis then we need to look at a cohort study. Equally if we have a research question we would like to investigate we need to use the most appropriate study design to answer that question (see Table 2-1).

2.5 Dental evidence base

So how much evidence do we have? Work conducted by Dr. R. Niederman at Harvard (1999) has compared the number of randomised controlled trials for different specialities in medicine with dentistry. Dentistry is a poor per-

2.5 Dental evidence base

Table 2-1: Appropriate study designs						
	Qualitative	Cross Sectional	Case Controlled	Cohort	RCT	Systematic Review
Diagnosis				☆	☆☆	☆☆☆
Therapy				☆	☆☆	☆☆☆
Prognosis				☆☆☆		
Screening			☆	☆	☆☆	☆☆☆
Views/beliefs perceptions	☆☆☆					
Managerial innovation	☆		☆	☆	☆☆	☆☆☆
Hypothesis generation	☆☆☆					
Prevalence		☆☆☆				

☆ The more stars the more appropriate the study design.

former in terms of the number of randomised controlled trials. If we look at specialities within dentistry we see that periodontologists carry out the most RCTs, with endodontists carrying out least.

A similar look at the evidence base for oral health was conducted in Wales (cf. Health Evidence Bulletins Wales, 1998) and it shows that much of our evidence-base rests with the lower grades of evidence (see Table 2-2).

So we could sum up the current evidence base of dentistry with this pie chart (see Fig. 2-3). The challenge is to move towards a point where all the interventions we perform are either known to do more good than harm or are else part of a properly conducted study (see Fig. 2-4).

"The fact that an opinion has been widely held is no evidence whatever that it is not utterly absurd; indeed in view of the silliness of the majority of mankind, a widespread belief is more likely to be foolish than sensible".

Bertrand Russell (1872–1970) in "Marriage and Morals" (1929), Ch. 5

Table 2-2: The evidence-base for oral health (from Health Evidence Bulletins Wales, 1998)

	Statements	Levels of supporting evidence[1]				
		I[2]	II	III	IV	V
Tooth Decay	26	9 (7)	0	8	4	17
Periodontal disease	14	13 (8)	0	1	1	2
Dento-facial anomalies	15	1	0	0	1	6
Oral Cancer	10	0	0	0	11	7
TMJ Disorders	7	0	0	1	0	6
Tooth Wear	12	0	0	0	10	4
Dental injuries	16	0	1	3	5	9
Inherited anomalies	7	0	0	0	1	7
Total	**107**	**23 (15)**	**1**	**13**	**33**	**58**

[1] Levels of evidence relate to the AHCPR grading with level I being the strongest and V the weakest
[2] Figures in brackets in level I are the actual number of systematic reviews, the higher is present as some reviews answer more than one statement.

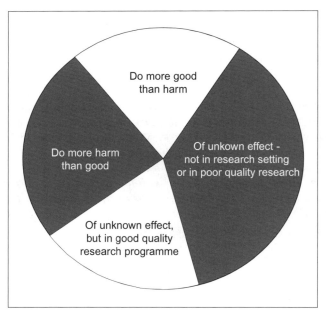

Figure 2-3: Estimate of the current position of the evidence-base of dental interventions

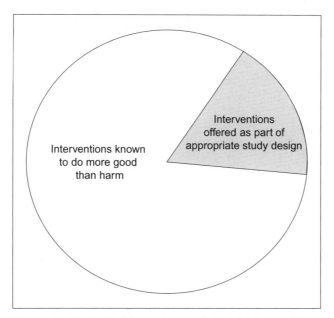

Figure 2-4: Future aim for the evidence-base of dental interventions

2.6 Users and doers

Although the title divides the scientist and the practitioner I feel that it is a false divide and the whole profession should have a "scientific approach". We can however identify two groups within the profession. The USERS of evidence, which should be the whole profession, and the researchers or DOERS.

The challenges for users are:
– to be able to formulate a question or questions from a patients presenting condition,
– to know which sources of evidence to use and how to access them,
– to be able to critically appraise the evidence they find,
– complain when information in scientific literature is badly presented/ poorly explained.

Dunn et al. (1997) found that 75% of nurses cannot understand the statistics with 70% being unable to critically appraise a research paper. While Vine and Hastings (1994) found that "Most doctors answer in the affirmative when asked whether they would take a daily pill to reduce their chances of dying from a heart attack by 50%." But, "When asked if they would do so for 10 to 20 years if the risk was reduced from 2/1000 to 1/1000, a reduction of 50%, there is much less enthusiasm!".

Table 2-3: Errors in study design	
	Percentage papers exhibiting problems
	%
Planning	5
Design	22
Execution	18
Data processing	5
Interpretation	6

The "doers" carry out basic research, which is essential for dentistry to progress and secondary research or systematic reviews, which are assuming greater importance. But Sackett (1979) found a wide range of problems with basic research (see Table 2-3). Schor and Karten (1966) found a worrying level of statistical problems in papers published in the journal of the American Medical Association, a fact that Altman (1991) found little improved some years later.

Mulrow (1987) examined 50 reviews in four major journals that appeared between 1985 and 1986. He found 49 had no statement of the methods involved with 47 having inappropriate summaries. He concluded, "Current medical reviews do not routinely use scientific methods to identify, assess and synthesise information."

Silagy (1993) looked at reviews in primary care journals and although there had been an improvement there is room for much greater change. In Dentistry I suspect, we are at best in the same position as Mulrow (1987) found in Medicine, but possibly worse off.

2.7 The challenges ahead

So we can identify a number of challenges for the dental profession:
− to be able to ask how to ask/set good questions,
− to know where to look for evidence,
− to be able to critical appraisal,
− to complain.

A number of challenges for Primary researchers:
− better training in research skills,
− greater awareness of appropriate research designs,
− better presentation and dissemination of results.

A number of challenges for Secondary researchers:
- more training in systematic review methodology,
- more systematic reviews,
- better dissemination.

2.8 Dissemination and implementation

Dissemination of good evidence is a problem. Two recent examples from the UK illustrate the point. Two major reviews of oral health promotion (cf. Sprod, Anderson and Treasure, 1966; Kay and Locker, 1998) have been carried out and yet the bulk of the profession when asked are not aware of them. Furthermore evidence-based guidelines on the use of radiographs in dental literature have received even less attention despite their development by the Faculty of General Dental Practitioners (1999).

This leads to implementation. This is probably the most challenging area yet much research has been done in this area and the most consistently effective strategies have been identified in a series of Cochrane review (cf. Bero et al., 1998). Those found to have the greatest effect are:

- educational outreach,
- reminders,
- interactive educational meetings,
- multifaceted interventions.

While those having the least effect are:
- educational materials,
- didactic educational meetings.

2.9 Conclusion

In summary the best health care is that which is based on the best available evidence, with all ineffective interventions eliminated; with the interventions undertaken being of highest possible effectiveness for those groups of patients most likely to benefit, and all services being delivered at the highest possible quality.

An evidence-based approach to dentistry can help achieve this. The approach can be summarised into five main points:

- Decisions should be made on best available evidence,
- Based on patients' clinical problem.
- Evidence should be integrated from all sources.
- Conclusions from critically appraised evidence must be clinically important.
- Professionals must continually appraise their performance.

It is however not new and most good practitioners have always practised in this way, and as if to prove my point I will now close with this quote which to me sums up the questioning approach that evidence-based methodology brings to dentistry:

"If a man will begin with certainties, he shall end in doubts; but if he will be content to begin with doubts, he shall end in certainties."
Francis Bacon (1561–1626) in "The Advancement of Learning" (1605)

You may like to note that it was written almost 400 years ago!

2.10 Literatur/References

AHCPR: US Department of Health and Human Services, Public Health Service, Agency Health Care Policy and Research. Acute Pain Management: Operative or Medical Procedures and Trauma. Agency for Health Care Policy and Research Publications, Rockville, MD. (AHCPR Pub 92-0038) 1992

Altman, D. G.: Statistics in medical journals: developments in the 1980s. Stat Med 10 (1991), 1897–1913

Bero, L. A., Grilli, R., Grimshaw, J. M., Harvey, E., Oxman, A. D., Thomson, M. A.: Closing the gap between research and practice: an overview of systematic reviews of interventions to promote the implementation of research findings. The Cochrane Effective Practise and Organization of Care Review Group. BMJ 317 (1998), 465-468

Dunn, V., Chrichton, C., Williams, K., Roe, B., Seers, K.: Using Research for Practice: A UK Experience of the BARRIERS scale. J Adv Nurs 26 (1997), 1203-1210

Faculty of General Dental Practitioners: Selection Criteria for Dental Radiography. UK, 1999

Health Evidence Bulletins Wales – Oral Health. March 1998 Iechyd Morgannwg Health. Team Leader Tony Glenn. NHS Cymru Wales (http://www.uwcm.ac.uk/uwcm/lb/pep/oralhealth/index.html)

Kay, E., Locker, D.: A systematic review of the effectiveness of health promotion aimed at promoting oral health. London: Health Education Authority, 1998

Mulrow, C. D.: The medical review article: state of the science. Ann Intern Med 106 (1987), 485–488

Niederman, R.: Persönl. Mitteilung/personal communication, Harvard 1999

Sackett, D. L.: Bias in analytic research. J Chronic Dis 32 (1979), 51–63

Sackett, D. L., Rosenberg, W. M., Gray, J. A., Haynes, R. B., Richardson, W. S.: Evidence based medicine: what it is and what it isn't. BMJ 312 (1996), 71–72

Schor, S., Karten, I.: Statistical evaluation of medical journal manuscripts. JAMA 195 (1966), 1123–1128

Shin, J. H., Haynes, R. B., Johnston, M. E.: Effect of problem-based, self-directed undergraduate education on life-long learning. Can Med Assoc J 148 (1993), 969–976

Silagy, C. A.: An analysis of review articles published in primary care journals. Fam Pract 10 (1993), 337–341

Sprod, A., Anderson, R., Treasure, E.: Effective oral health promotion. Literature review. Cardiff, Wales: Health Promotion Wales, 1996; Technical report

Vine, D. L., Hastings, G.: Ischaemic heart disease and cholesterol. Absolute risk more informative than relative risk. BMJ 308 (1994), 1040–1041

3 Evidenz-basierte Medizin – die Suche und Anwendung von gesicherten Entscheidungsgrundlagen

Matthias Perleth, Hannover

3.1 Einleitung: Anmerkungen zum Evidenzbegriff

In der Medizin lassen sich mehrere Evidenzbegriffe voneinander abgrenzen. Hierzu gehören unter anderem ein juristischer, biomedizinischer, klinisch-praktischer und ein methodischer Evidenzbegriff. Im Folgenden werden diese unterschiedlichen Betrachtungsweisen kurz erläutert.

Der juristische Begriff von Evidenz bezieht sich auf das, was vor Gericht als Beweismaterial zugelassen wird. Problematisch hierbei ist der uneinheitliche Umgang mit dem Begriff der Evidenz. Bei Erstattungsentscheidungen der Sozialgerichte, die vermeintlich im Sinne der Patienten gefällt werden, verschwimmt bisweilen die Grenze zwischen Scharlatanerie und Seriosität. Andererseits definiert Hart (1998) bezogen auf die klinische Medizin einen Standard als die in der wissenschaftlichen Literatur feststellbare Evidenz in Verbindung mit ärztlicher Erfahrung und professioneller Akzeptanz. In der biomedizinischen Definition gilt als Evidenz, was sich pathophysiologisch plausibel erklären bzw. vorhersagen lässt. Klinisch-praktisch reicht oft die klinische Erfahrung von Ärzten in Kombination mit Einzelstudien als Evidenz aus. Der methodische Evidenzbegriff fokussiert auf die durch systematische Suche und Datensynthese möglichst objektiv und vollständig erfassbare Datenlage und ohne Präferenz für pathophysiologische Zusammenhänge.

Die Wirksamkeit einer Maßnahme kann in mehreren Dimensionen betrachtet werden. Wenn an der Effektivität einer Technologie unter definierten (experimentellen) Bedingungen kein Zweifel besteht, die Wirkung also offensichtlich ist, dann sind auch keine aufwendigen Studien zum Nachweis der Wirksamkeit notwendig (vgl. Abb. 3-1). So bedarf es zum Beispiel keiner aufwendigen Studien, um zu zeigen, dass unkomplizierte Knochenbrüche – eine lege-artis-Behandlung vorausgesetzt – durch Einrichten und Eingipsen erfolgreich behandelt werden können.

Aufwendigere und genauere Methoden zum Nachweis der Wirkung werden notwendig, je weniger eindeutig die Effektivität einer Maßnahme ist. Aller-

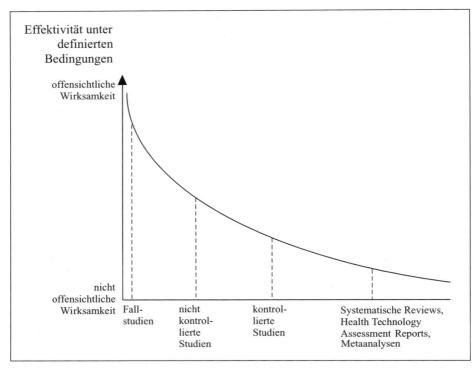

Abbildung 3-1: Zusammenhang zwischen Wirksamkeit und Instrumenten zum Nachweis der Wirksamkeit

dings ist die Effektivität abhängig von einer Reihe von Faktoren, die oft eine eindeutige Beurteilung erschweren. Hierzu gehören u. a.: Gesundheit der Patienten vor der Intervention; Art der Krankheit und Prognose; lokal verfügbare Therapieoptionen; Fähigkeiten und Qualifikationen der Leistungserbringer (vgl. Abb. 3-1).

3.2 Was versteht man unter „gesicherter Evidenz"?

Eine einheitliche Definition von gesicherter Evidenz ist nicht möglich, da die Anforderungen an das Studiendesign je nach Fragestellung erheblich voneinander abweichen können. Fallstudien beispielsweise können durchaus von Nutzen sein, etwa um ein bisher nicht beachtetes Problem zu beleuchten, Forschungsfragen zu generieren oder Hypothesen zu widerlegen. Insofern ist die Frage der Adäquanz voranzustellen. Zunächst sollte also geprüft werden, ob ein klinisches Problem überhaupt methodisch sinnvoll in Angriff genommen wurde. Hierzu gehört nicht nur die Auswahl eines geeigneten Designs, sondern auch die Beachtung biometrischer Grundregeln, etwa eine geeignete Stichprobengröße.

Der Goldstandard für therapeutische Fragestellungen ist die randomisierte kontrollierte Studie. Für prognostische Fragestellungen sind eher Kohortenstudien geeignet, in der eine Gruppe von Personen (Kohorte) mit einer bestimmten Krankheit oder einer Exposition mit einer anderen Gruppe ohne dieses Merkmal über einen längeren Zeitraum hinsichtlich des Auftretens einer Zielerkrankung verglichen wird. Idealerweise befinden sich alle Patienten im gleichen Krankheitsstadium. Diagnostische Studien sollten folgende Kriterien erfüllen: randomisierte Zuordnung aller Patienten zu allen Untersuchungsmethoden, verblindet durchgeführter Vergleich mit diagnostischem Goldstandard, Anwendung bei einem breiten Patientenspektrum (gemäß klinischer Routinebedingungen), Angabe von Wahrscheinlichkeitsverhältnissen für positive und negative Testresultate. Dies kann mit unterschiedlichen Studiendesigns erreicht werden.

Sind diese Voraussetzungen erfüllt, dann ist zu klären, ob und wie viele Studien zu einer Fragestellung vorhanden sind. Es gibt keine allgemeingültigen Antworten auf die Frage, wie viele Studien vorliegen müssen, um von gesicherter Evidenz sprechen zu können. Bei prognostischen Fragestellungen kann u. U. eine einzige Kohortenstudie ausreichen, um eine definitive Aussage machen zu können. Für therapeutische Fragestellungen liegen oft mehrere Studien vor, die erfahrungsgemäß Unterschiede in Design, eingeschlossener Patientenpopulation, Wahl der Ergebnisparameter usw. aufweisen. Problematisch ist die Situation dann, wenn vom Design her vergleichbare Studien zu unterschiedlichen Aussagen kommen. Es gibt Beispiele in der Literatur, wie durch selektives Zitieren von Studien, welche die eigene Hypothese stützen, und gleichzeitiges Ignorieren von gegensinnigen Studien verzerrte Aussagen getroffen wurden (vgl. z. B. Knipschild, 1994).

Systematische Übersichten (Reviews) sind definiert als Übersichten einer klar formulierten Fragestellung, bei der systematisch und anhand expliziter Kriterien relevante Literatur identifiziert, selektiert und bewertet und qualitativen Analysen und eventuell einer quantitativen Analyse (Meta-Analyse) unterzogen wird (vgl. Tab. 3-1). Sie sind das derzeit beste Instrument, um die vorhandene Evidenz zusammenzufassen. Demnach kann als gesicherte Evidenz gelten, wenn ein systematischer Review die einer Fragestellung angemessenen Studien in möglichst hoher Qualität und mit möglichst gleichsinnigen Aussagen (= Homogenität) vollständig erfasst hat und so zu einer unverzerrten Aussage des an den wahren Wert approximierten Ergebnisses kommt.

Systematische Reviews sind von sogenannten narrativen Reviews abzugrenzen (vgl. Tab. 3-2), die traditionell ein großes Wissensgebiet, oft auch aus der Grundlagenforschung, behandeln, aufgrund ihrer nicht systematischen Anlage aber zu verzerrten Aussagen kommen können.

Tabelle 3-1: Komponenten der systematischen Übersicht

Komponente	Beispiel (Perleth, Jakubowski und Busse, 1999)
fokussierte und eindeutige Fragestellung	Wie groß ist die Anzahl und Qualität der Studien zu verschiedenen diagnostischen Methoden der akuten Sinusitis maxillaris bei Erwachsenen und wie sind die unterschiedlichen diagnostischen Verfahren hinsichtlich ihrer diagnostischen Wertigkeit relativ zueinander zu bewerten?
Formulierung von Ein- und Ausschlusskriterien	Primärstudien, die mindestens zwei diagnostische Verfahren bei Patienten über 15 Jahre mit Symptomen der akuten Sinusitis maxillaris und einer Symptomdauer <3 Monate verglichen
vollständige Identifikation relevanter Studien	22 Primärstudien (mit insgesamt 40 Vergleichen) sowie drei Leitlinien und zwei Meta-Analysen wurden eingeschlossen
Qualitätsbewertung gefundener Studien	Bewertung der methodischen Qualität sowie Einordnung in die jeweilige Evaluationsphase
standardisierte Auswertung	Die Daten wurden von zwei Untersuchern unabhängig voneinander in Vierfeldertafeln extrahiert und bei Differenzen abgeglichen
Synthese, qualitativ oder quantitativ	Darstellung in Tabellen und, wo angemessen, in Meta-Analysen

Tabelle 3-2: Unterschiede zwischen narrativen und systematischen Übersichten

Merkmal	Narrativer Review	Systematischer Review
Frage	oft breit angelegt	fokussierte klinische Fragestellung
Literatursuche	meist nicht angegeben, Gefahr des „publication bias"	umfangreiche Recherche, explizite Suchstrategie
Auswahl der Studien	meist nicht angegeben, Gefahr des bias	auf vorher festgelegten Kriterien basierend, bei allen Studien angewandt
Bewertung der Studien	variabel	auf Kriterien basiert, bei allen Studien angewandt
Synthese	meist qualitative Zusammenfassung	oft Meta-Analyse
Schlussfolgerungen	manchmal evidenz-basiert	meist evidenz-basiert, Abstufung entsprechend Evidenzhierarchie
Aktualisierung	selten	oft

3.3 Die Cochrane Collaboration

Weltweit schrittmachend und den methodischen Standard für systematische Übersichten vorgebend ist die Cochrane Collaboration. Die Cochrane Collaboration ist ein internationales Netzwerk von Ärzten mit dem Ziel der Erstellung und periodischen Aktualisierung systematischer Übersichten von vorzugsweise randomisierten kontrollierten Studien in allen relevanten Bereichen der medizinischen Versorgung und deren Bereitstellung für Entscheidungsträger auf allen Ebenen des Gesundheitswesens.

Das Logo der Cochrane Collaboration (vgl. Abb. 3-2) zeigt das Ergebnis einer systematischen Übersicht. Der Diamant zeigt den Effekt einer kurzdauernden Kortisontherapie bei drohender Frühgeburt. Die 7 Studien von 1972 bis 1982 zeigen eine um 30–50% höhere Überlebenschance Frühgeborener. Erst ab 1989 wurde die Effektivität dieser Maßnahme aber allgemein bekannt und gebräuchlich. Dieser Aspekt zeigt aber auch, dass mit der jeweils verfügbaren Methodik immer nur begrenzte Aussagen möglich sind. Zu Beginn der 1980er-Jahre waren Meta-Analysen in der Medizin beispielsweise noch nicht verbreitet.

3.4 Das Problem der Generalisierbarkeit

Zu beachten ist in diesem Zusammenhang die Frage der Generalisierbarkeit, vor allem therapeutischer Studien. Therapiestudien – insbesondere randomisierte kontrollierte Studien – werden oft unter idealen Bedingungen, meist in Universitätskliniken mit hochmotivierten Ärzten und streng selektierten Patienten, durchgeführt. Die unter diesen Umständen gewonnenen Resultate bezeichnet man als Effektivität unter Idealbedingungen (,efficacy'). Dem steht die unter alltäglichen Bedingungen erreichbare Wirksamkeit einer medizinischen Intervention gegenüber (,effectiveness').

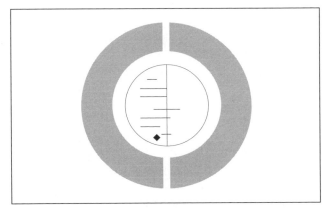

Abbildung 3-2: Logo der Cochrane Collaboration

Ioannidis und Lau (1997) haben in einer Untersuchung zur Generalisierbarkeit von Therapiestudien den möglichen Einfluss der Auswahl der Studienteilnehmer auf die Studienergebnisse untersucht. Sie verglichen dabei die Verteilung des Ausgangsrisikos verschiedener Studienpopulationen für einen binären Endpunkt (hier: Einfluss der Magnesiumgabe auf die Herzinfarktmortalität), das entsprechend den Einschlusskriterien modelliert wurde.

Die Ergebnisse von kleinen klinischen Studien, die heterogene Populationen mit binären Endpunkten untersuchen, hängen oft von den Resultaten von wenigen Hochrisikopatienten ab. Umgekehrt können große Studien mit homogenen Studienpopulationen Subgruppen oder Individuen mit hohem Risiko oder untypischen Therapieantworten ausschließen. In beiden Fällen kann die unkritische Aggregierung der Daten zu Fehlinterpretationen führen.

Die Überrepräsentierung von Hochrisikogruppen oder die Präsenz noch unbekannter Risikofaktoren kann die Verallgemeinerbarkeit von Studienergebnissen einschränken. Diese Vorbehalte sind insbesondere dann von Bedeutung, wenn der Nutzen einer Therapie nicht über das gesamte Spektrum von Ausgangsrisiken gleich ist. Die Autoren plädieren deshalb für eine Prästratifizierung von Patienten vor dem Studieneinschluss nach ihrem jeweiligem Risikoprofil (vgl. Abb. 3-3).

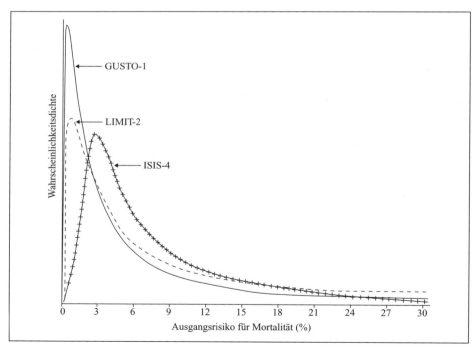

Abbildung 3-3: Risikoverteilung in verschiedenen Studien
Quelle: Ionnidis und Lau, 1997

3.4 Das Problem der Generalisierbarkeit

Die Modellierung der Konsequenzen von therapeutischen Studien zur Magnesiumgabe bei akutem Herzinfarkt soll hier kurz dargestellt werden. Dabei wurden im Wesentlichen die Ergebnisse von drei Studien-Modellen (ISIS-4, GUSTO-I, LIMIT-2) miteinander verglichen. Die GUSTO-I-Studie lieferte für das Modell das Profil einer heterogenen Studienpopulation, in der 10% der Hochrisikopatienten die Hälfte der Gesamtmortalität beitrugen. ISIS-4 schloss Patienten mit sehr hohem und sehr niedrigem Risiko aus, mit dem Ergebnis einer relativ homogenen Population. Die LIMIT-2-Studie umfasste eine heterogene Studienpopulation mit einem höheren durchschnittlichen Ausgangsrisiko (14% der Patienten trugen zwei Drittel der Gesamtmortalität bei) als GUSTO-I.

Die ‚effectiveness domain'

In einer eher theoretischen Betrachtung kann man eine sogenannte ‚effectiveness domain' konstruieren, das ist ein hypothetischer Evidenzraum, in dem für sämtliche Patientengruppen und für sämtliche Krankheitsstadien und für alle in Frage kommenden therapeutischen Alternativen die jeweils verfügbare Evidenz zusammengefasst ist. Ein stark vereinfachtes Beispiel einer ‚effectiveness domain' zeigt Abbildung 3-4.

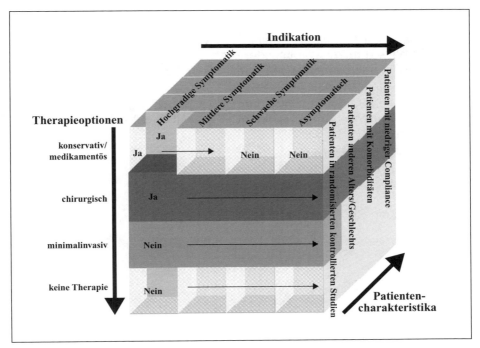

Abbildung 3-4: „Effectiveness Domain"

In diesem Beispiel sind Daten aus Studien zur Therapie der Karotisstenose bei symptomatisch und bei asymptomatisch erkrankten Patienten (horizontale Achse) zusammengestellt. Auf der vertikalen Achse sind die Therapieoptionen und auf der Z-Achse verschiedene Patientenprofile abgetragen. Dieses stark vereinfachte Schema zeigt, wie viele Einzelinformationen notwendig sind, um einen Überblick über die beste Therapiemöglichkeit bei gegebenen Patientencharakteristika und Krankheitsstadien zu erhalten. Die Informationen können aus klinischen Studien, Registern, administrativen Datenbanken und aus qualitativen Studien kommen (vgl. Jakubowski, Busse und Perleth, 1998).

3.5 Quellen für systematische Übersichten

Es gibt eine Reihe von wichtigen Quellen, die bei der systematischen Literatursuche im Vordergrund stehen sollten (vgl. Antes, 1997):

I   Cochrane Library (http://www.cochrane.de)
    – Systematische Reviews
    – Klassische Reviews
    – Literaturdatenbank zu kontrollierten klinischen Studien
    – Liste von Artikeln zur Methodik

IIa Literaturdatenbanken(systeme), Beispiele
    – Medline (http://www.dimdi.de/germ/fr-rech.htm, kostenlos)
    – HealthStar (http://igm-01.nlm.nih.gov/index.html, kostenlos)
    – Embase (http://www.dimdi.de, kostenpflichtig)
    – DIMDI (simultan mehrere Datenbanken, kostenminimierter Zugriff)

IIb Nutzerfreundliche Sekundärliteratur
    – Evidence-Based Dentistry (http://www.ihs.ox.ac.uk/cebd/ebdj.htm)
    – Best Evidence auf CD-ROM: ACP Journal Club/Evidence-Based Medicine

III Spezielle Datenbanken
    – von Forschergruppen
    – Register klinischer Studien

Nachfolgend ein Recherche-Beispiel:

> **Beispiel: Recherche von kontrollierten Studien und Reviews/Meta-Analysen im Bereich der Zahnmedizin**
>
> Recherche in der Cochrane Library, Version 4/99, nur RCTs und CCTs:
>
> - Stichworte: dental* and (prostheses-and-implants*:ME)
>   299 Treffer seit 1990, davon 2 Meta-Analysen, 2 systematische Übersichten und 295 RCTs und CCTs
> - Suche in MEDLINE und HealthStar nach Übersichtsarbeiten:
>   2 Meta-Analysen und 279 Reviews seit 1992
>
> Die Studien (RCTs *und* CCTs) verteilten sich prozentual auf die folgenden Bereiche:
>
> | | |
> |---|---|
> | Füllungen | 23% |
> | Implantate | 26% |
> | Karies | 11% |
> | Arzneimittel | 9% |
> | Kronen | 5% |
> | Zahnersatz | 11% |
> | sonstige Studien (inklusive Parodontalerkrankungen) | 15% |

3.6 Anwendungskontext und Ausblick

Wer profitiert von systematischen Reviews?

Systematische Reviews, die hohe Qualitätsanforderungen erfüllen, können Entscheidungen auf allen Ebenen des Gesundheitswesens unterstützen. Hier sind vor allem folgende Ebenen von Bedeutung: Kliniker, Selbstverwaltungsgremien und Patienten.

Für die Klinik haben systematische Übersichten eine zunehmende Bedeutung. Hierauf deuten Ergebnisse einer Umfrage bei australischen Neonatologen und Geburtshelfern (vgl. Jordens et al., 1998) hin: 21% gaben spontan an, systematische Reviews gezielt zu verwenden. Auf Nachfrage nutzten 72% der Neonatologen und 44% der Geburtshelfer systematische Reviews. Zugang zu entsprechenden Datenbanken sowie Vertrautheit von Computern waren entscheidende Voraussetzungen für deren Nutzung. 58% der Neonatologen und 80% der Geburtshelfer, die auf systematische Reviews zurückgreifen, gaben an, dass diese ihre Praxis beeinflussen. Diese aus dem Jahr 1995 stammenden Ergebnisse dürften heute noch besser zugunsten von systematischen Reviews ausfallen.

Ein weiterer wichtiger Bereich sind Investitionen im Krankenhausbereich. Insbesondere in den USA hat sich eine Unternehmenskultur etabliert, die auf die systematische Bewertung einer Technologie zurückgreift, bevor umfangreiche Investitionen vorgenommen werden (vgl. Rettig, 1997).

In Deutschland nimmt die systematische Bewertung medizinischer Verfahren im Rahmen der Selbstverwaltung einen immer größeren Stellenwert ein. Hier ist besonders der Bundesausschuss der Ärzte und Krankenkassen zu erwähnen, dessen Arbeitsausschuss Ärztliche Behandlung zunehmend auf systematische Übersichten zurückgreift (Perleth, Busse und Schwartz, 1999). Im Bundesausschuss der Zahnärzte und Krankenkassen hat sich ebenfalls ein entsprechender Arbeitsausschuss etabliert.

Auch für Patienten werden systematische Reviews zugänglich gemacht. Ein Beispiel ist das von einer deutschen Krankenkasse zur Verfügung gestellte evidenz-basierte Patienteninformationssystem im Internet (www.therapie.net). Als Basis der Patienteninformationen dienen wissenschaftliche, systematische Übersichtsarbeiten, die den aktuellen internationalen Informationsstand zur Wirksamkeit und zu Risiken ausgewählter Therapie- und Diagnoseverfahren wiedergeben und bewerten. Auf dieser Grundlage werden allgemein verständliche Laieninformationen erstellt, wobei – internationalen Qualitätskriterien folgend – die Informationsbedürfnisse der potentiellen Nutzer im Vordergrund stehen, z. B.: Informationen über die jeweilige Erkrankung, ihre Verbreitung sowie Risikofaktoren und Vorbeugemaßnahmen; Ziel, Durchführung, Dauer des beschriebenen Verfahrens; Nutzen und Risiken; alternative Möglichkeiten (vgl. Reichle und Lerch, 1999).

Es ist zu erwarten, dass systematische Übersichten in Zukunft einen größeren Stellenwert erlangen und auch stärker für andere als therapeutische Fragestellungen (Diagnostik, Epidemiologie) Anwendung finden. Als universelles Instrument können sie in unterschiedlichen Anwendungskontexten eingesetzt werden, wie z. B. Leitlinienentwicklung, Technologiebewertung, Patienteninformation und vor allem als Beitrag zur klinischen Entscheidungsfindung.

3 Evidence-based medicine: seeking and applying reliable foundations for decision-making

Matthias Perleth, Hannover

3.1 Introduction: Notes on the concept of evidence

Several different concepts of evidence can be distinguished from each other in medicine – for example in the legal and biomedical fields and in those of clinical practice and methodology. These various approaches will be briefly elucidated in this paper.

As a legal term, evidence means what is admissible as testimony in court. One problem here is the lack of standardization in regard to the term's use. In decisions by the German Social Courts on reimbursement, which are notionally made for patients' benefit, the boundary between charlatanism and serious professional practice is sometimes blurred. Hart (1998), on the other hand, defines a standard, in relation to clinical medicine, as the evidence to be found in the scientific literature coupled with medical experience and professional acceptance. For biomedical purposes, evidence is defined as something that can be plausibly explained or, as the case may be, predicted pathophysiologically. In clinical practice, the clinical experience of doctors together with individual studies often suffices as evidence. The methodological concept of evidence focuses on the data determinable as objectively and comprehensively as possible by systematic searching and synthesis of all the relevant information, without according preference to pathophysiological connections.

The effectiveness of a measure can be considered on several different levels. If there is no doubt about the efficacy of a technology under defined (experimental) conditions – i.e. if the effect is manifest – complicated and expensive studies to demonstrate it are unnecessary (see Fig. 3-1). For example, there is no need for such studies in order to show that simple fractures can – assuming therapy performed with due professional competence – be treated successfully by setting and encasement in plaster.

The less obvious it is that a measure is effective, the more complex and exact will be the methods required to prove effectiveness. However, effi-

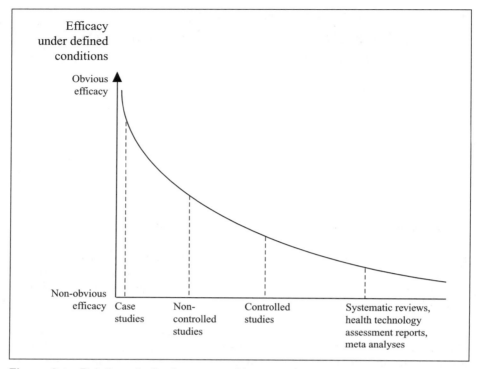

Figure 3-1: Relation of effectiveness and instruments for its demonstration

cacy depends on a number of factors that often make an unambiguous assessment difficult. These include, for instance, patients' general health before the intervention; the nature of the pathology and the prognosis; locally available therapy options; and the practitioners' skills and qualifications (see Fig. 3-1).

3.2 What is meant by "reliable evidence"?

It is not possible to give a standardized definition of reliable evidence, as the requirements to be satisfied by the study design will vary substantially from situation to situation. Case studies, for example, may perfectly well be useful for casting light on a hitherto unconsidered problem, generating research topics or refuting hypotheses. From this point of view, the question of appropriateness must be asked first. Hence the first step should be to examine whether a clinical problem can reasonably be tackled by a methodological approach at all. This involves not only the choice of a suitable design but also the observance of basic biometric rules, such as appropriate random sample size.

3.2 What is meant by "reliable evidence"?

The gold standard for questions of therapy is the randomized controlled study. Where the issue is prognosis, cohort studies will be more suitable: here a group of subjects (a cohort) with a given condition or exposure is compared with another group lacking this attribute over a relatively long period in regard to the occurrence of a target disease. Ideally, all patients will be at the same stage of the condition. Diagnostic studies should meet the following criteria: randomized assignment of all patients to all investigative methods; blind comparison with the diagnostic gold standard; use with a wide range of patients (under routine clinical conditions); and statement of probabilities for positive and negative test results. This can be achieved with different study designs.

If these conditions are satisfied, the next step is to determine whether any studies exist on the relevant topic, and, if so, how many. There is no universally valid answer to the question of the number of studies required in order for the evidence to be deemed reliable. For problems involving prognosis, a single cohort study may sometimes suffice to permit a definitive statement. Where therapy is concerned there are often a number of studies, which, as experience shows, are likely to differ in design, included patient population, choice of result parameters, and so on. Problems arise when studies of comparable design yield different results. Examples in the literature show how results have been distorted by an author's selective citation of studies that support his own hypothesis while ignoring others that conflict with it (e.g. Knipschild, 1994).

Systematic reviews are defined as reviews of a clearly defined problem situation in which a systematic approach involving explicit criteria is used to identify, select and assess relevant literature and to subject it to qualitative and possibly also quantitative analysis (meta-analysis) (see Table 3-1). They are at present the best instrument we have for synthesizing the available evidence. On this basis, evidence may be deemed reliable where a systematic review has comprehensively covered the studies relevant to a given subject at as high as possible a quality level and with as homogeneous as possible results, thus leading to an undistorted end-result approximating to the true value of the parameters concerned.

Systematic reviews must be distinguished from "narrative reviews" (see Table 3-2), which traditionally cover a broad field of knowledge, often also including fundamental research, but may yield distorted results owing to their non-systematic design.

Table 3-1: Components of a systematic review

Component	Example (cf. Perleth, Jakubowski and Busse, 1999)
Focused and unequivocally defined topic	How many studies have been conducted on various diagnostic methods for acute maxillary sinusitis in adults, what is the quality of these studies, and how are the various diagnostic techniques to be rated relative to each other in terms of their diagnostic value?
Formulation of criteria for inclusion and exclusion	Primary studies comparing at least two diagnostic methods in patients aged over 15 years with symptoms of acute maxillary sinusitis of less than three months' duration
Complete identification of relevant studies	22 primary studies (with a total of 40 comparisons), three guidelines and two meta-analyses were included
Quality assessment of studies found	Assessment of methodological quality and assignment to the relevant phase of evaluation
Standardized evaluation	Data extracted independently by two research workers in two by two tables and a consent was sought in the event of discrepancies
Synthesis, qualitative or quantitative	Presentation in tables and, where appropriate, in meta-analyses

Table 3-2: Differences between narrative and systematic reviews

Aspect	Narrative review	Systematic review
Subject matter	often broadly based	focused clinical topic
Literature search	not usually specified; risk of publication bias	extensive searching; explicit search strategy
Selection of studies	not usually stated; risk of bias	based on predetermined criteria used for all studies
Assessment of studies	variable	based on criteria applied to all studies
Synthesis	usually qualitative	often meta-analysis
Conclusions	sometimes evidence-based	usually evidence-based; graded by hierarchy of evidence
Updated	seldom	frequently

3.3 The Cochrane Collaboration

The Cochrane Collaboration is a worldwide pacemaker that sets the methodological standard for systematic reviews. It is an international network of doctors that exists to compile and periodically update systematic reviews of preferably randomized controlled studies in all relevant fields of medical care and to make them available to decision-makers at all levels of the health system.

The logo of the Cochrane Collaboration (see Fig. 3-2) represents the result of a systematic review. The diamond shows the effect of short-term cortisone therapy in a patient at risk of giving birth prematurely. The seven studies from the period 1972 to 1982 show that such premature babies have a 30–50% higher probability of survival. However, it was only from 1989 that this measure came to be generally known and used. This example also shows that only limited statements can be made on the basis of the methodology available at any given time. For instance, meta-analyses were not yet in common use in medicine in the early 1980s.

3.4 The problem of generalizability

The issue of generalizability, especially in regard to therapeutic studies, is relevant in this connection. Therapeutic studies – in particular, randomized controlled studies – are often carried out under ideal conditions, usually at university clinics with highly motivated doctors and strictly selected patients. The results obtained in these circumstances are described as "efficacy". This contrasts with the "effectiveness" of a medical intervention achievable under everyday conditions.

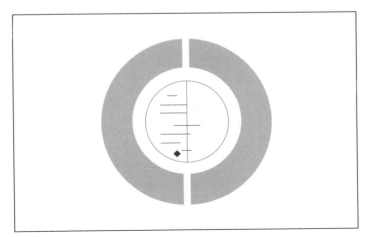

Figure 3-2: Logo of the Cochrane Collaboration

In an examination of the generalizability of therapeutic studies, Ioannidis and Lau (1997) investigated the possible influence of the choice of subjects on the results of a study. They here compared the distribution of the initial risk of different study populations for a binary end-point (in this case, the effect of magnesium administration on mortality from cardiac infarction), modelled in accordance with the inclusion criteria.

The results of small-scale clinical studies of heterogeneous populations with binary end-points often depend on the outcome in the cases of a small number of high-risk patients. Conversely, large-scale studies of homogeneous populations may exclude subgroups or individuals with high risks or atypical responses to therapy. Uncritical aggregation of the data may lead to misinterpretation in both cases.

Over-representation of high-risk groups or the presence of as yet unknown risk factors may limit the generalizability of study results. These reservations are important especially where the benefits of a therapy are not uniform over the entire spectrum of initial risks. The authors therefore advocate prestratification of patients by individual risk profile before inclusion in a study (see Fig. 3-3).

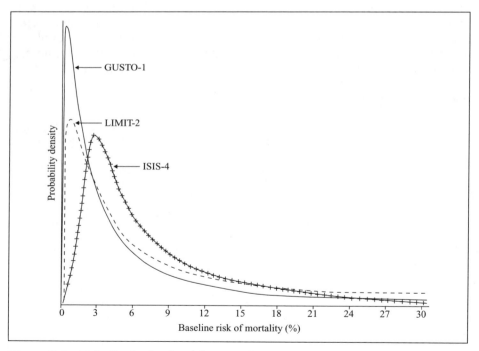

Figure 3-3: Risk distribution in various studies
Source: Ionnidis & Lau, 1997

3.4 The problem of generalizability

The modelling of the consequences of therapeutic studies on the administration of magnesium in cases of acute cardiac infarction will now be briefly described. The description is based mainly on a comparison of the results of three study models (ISIS-4, GUSTO-I and LIMIT-2). The GUSTO-I study supplied the model with the profile of a heterogeneous study population in which 10% of the high-risk patients accounted for half the total mortality. ISIS-4 excluded patients with very high and very low risks, so that the population was relatively homogeneous. The LIMIT-2 study covered a heterogeneous population with a higher average initial risk than in GUSTO-I (14% of the patients account for two thirds of total mortality).

The effectiveness domain

Considering the situation more from the theoretical standpoint, we can construct an "effectiveness domain" – i.e. a hypothetical evidential space that contains the whole of the relevant available evidence for all patient groups, all stages of the disease and all potentially applicable alternative forms of therapy. A highly simplified example of an effectiveness domain is given in Figure 3-4.

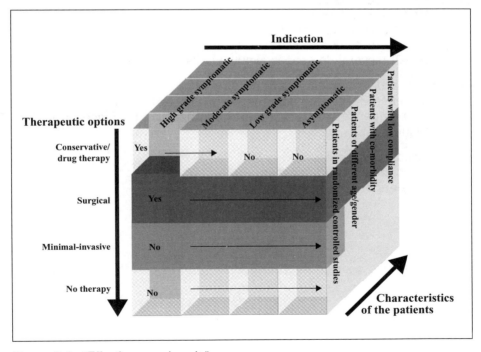

Figure 3-4: "Effectiveness domain"

In this example, data from studies on the therapy of carotid artery stenosis in patients both with and without symptoms are plotted along the horizontal axis. The vertical axis represents therapeutic options, while different patient profiles appear on the Z-axis. This highly simplified diagram shows how many individual items of information are necessary for an overview of the optimum therapies for given patient characteristics and stages in the pathological process. The information may be obtained from clinical studies, registers, administrative databases and qualitative studies (cf. Jakubowski, Busse and Perleth, 1998).

3.5 Sources for systematic reviews

There are a number of important sources that ought to feature prominently in any systematic literature search (cf. Antes, 1997):

I   Cochrane Library (http://www.cochrane.de)
- Systematic reviews
- Classical reviews
- Literature database of controlled clinical studies
- List of articles on methodology

IIa Literature databases and database systems (examples)
- Medline (http://www.dimdi.de/germ/fr-rech.htm, free)
- HealthStar (http://igm-01.nlm.nih.gov/index.html, free)
- Embase (http://www.dimdi.de, chargeable)
- DIMDI (several databases simultaneously, cost-minimized access)

IIb User-friendly secondary literature
- Evidence-Based Dentistry (http://www.ihs.ox.ac.uk/cebd/ebdj.htm)
- Best Evidence on CD-ROM: ACP Journal Club/Evidence-Based Medicine

III Specific databases
- research groups' databases
- registers of clinical studies

Example: search for controlled studies, reviews and meta-analyses in dentistry

Search in the Cochrane Library, version 4/99, RCTs and CCTs only:
− Keywords: dental* and (prostheses-and-implants*:ME)
  299 hits since 1990 (2 meta-analyses, 2 systematic reviews, 295 RCTs and CCTs)
− Search in MEDLINE and HealthStar for reviews:
  2 meta-analyses and 279 reviews since 1992
 	
Percentage breakdown of study topics:
 	
Fillings   23%
Implants   26%
Caries   11%
Medicines   9%
Crowns   5%
Prostheses   11%
Other studies (including periodontal diseases)   15%

3.6 Utilization context and outlook

Who benefits from systematic reviews?

High-quality systematic reviews can support decisions at all levels of the health-care system – in particular, by clinicians, self-governing committees and patients themselves.

Systematic reviews are becoming increasingly important for clinical practice. This is indicated by the results of a survey of Australian neonatologists and obstetricians (cf. Jordens et al., 1998), in which 21% of respondents spontaneously claimed to make specifically directed use of systematic reviews. When asked, 72% of the neonatologists and 44% of the obstetricians said they used systematic reviews. Access to relevant databases and familiarity with computers were crucial conditions for their use. 58% of the neonatologists and 80% of the obstetricians using systematic reviews stated that they influenced their practice. These results date from 1995; systematic reviews would surely fare even better today.

Capital investment in the hospital sector is another important field. In the United States in particular, a corporate-style culture that undertakes systematic evaluation of a technology prior to any large-scale investment has taken root (cf. Rettig, 1997).

The systematic evaluation of medical techniques in the context of self-government is assuming growing importance in Germany. Here the Bundesausschuss der Ärzte und Krankenkassen [Federal Committee of Physicians and Sick Funds] is worthy of particular mention: its Medical Treatment Subcommittee is making increasing use of systematic reviews (cf. Perleth, Busse and Schwartz, 1999). An equivalent subcommittee has been set up by the Bundesausschuss der Zahnärzte und Krankenkassen [Federal Committee of Dentists and Sick Funds].

Systematic reviews are made accessible to patients too. An example is the evidence-based patient information system made available by a German sick fund on the Internet (www.therapie.net). The patient information is based on scientific systematic reviews which reflect and assess the latest international consensus on the effectiveness and risks of selected therapeutic and diagnostic methods. This provides the foundation for the provision of information to lay persons in ordinary language; the prime concern here, in accordance with international quality criteria, is to satisfy the information needs of potential users on, for example, the relevant disease entity, its prevalence, risk factors and preventive measures; the object, conduct and duration of the treatment described; benefits and risks; and alternative possibilities (cf. Reichle and Lerch, 1999).

Systematic reviews are expected to gain significance in the future. This applies not only to therapeutic questions but also to other areas such as diagnosis and epidemiological problems. As universal instruments, systematic reviews may also be used in other contexts, for example development of clinical guidelines, health technology assessment or patient information systems and, of course, as aids to clinical decision-making.

3.7 Literatur/References

Antes, G.: EBM praktizieren. Wie erhalte ich Antwort auf meine Fragen? Münch med Wschr 139 (1997), 685–688

Hart, D.: Ärztliche Leitlinien – Definitionen, Funktionen, rechtliche Bewertungen. Gleichzeitig ein Beitrag zum medizinischen und rechtlichen Standardbegriff. MedR 16 (1998), 8–16

Ioannidis, J. P. A., Lau, J.: The impact of high-risk patients on the results of clinical trials. J Clin Epidemiol 50 (1997), 1089-1098

Jakubowski, E., Busse, R., Perleth, M.: Decision-making for 'Best Practice' in health care: The case of carotid endarterectomy. Annu Meet Int Soc Technol Assess Health Care 14 (1998), 66

Jordens, C. F., Hawe, P., Irwig, L. M., Henderson-Smart, D. J., Ryan, M., Donoghue, D. A., Gabb, R. G., Fraser, I. S.: Use of systematic reviews of randomised trials by Australian neonatologists and obstetricians. Med J Aust 168 (1998), 267–270

Knipschild, P.: Systematic Reviews: Some examples. BMJ 309 (1994), 719–721

Perleth, M., Busse, R., Schwartz, F. W.: Regulation of health-related technologies in Germany. Health Policy 46 (1999), 105–126

Perleth, M., Jakubowski, E., Busse, R.: Bewertung von Verfahren zur Diagnostik der akuten Sinusitis maxillaris bei Erwachsenen. Schriftenreihe Health Technology Assessment, Band 11, Baden-Baden, 1999

Reichle, C., Lerch, M.: Mehr Kompetenz durch evidenz-basierte Informationen im Internet. Public Health Forum 26 (1999), 18

Rettig, R. A.: Health care in transition. Technology assessment in the private sector, Santa Monica: RAND, 1997

4 Evidenz-basierte und patientenorientierte Medizin – zwei Modelle und ihr Zusammenhang

Jörg Michael Herrmann, Glottertal
Thure von Uexküll, Freiburg

4.1 Vorbemerkung: Zwei Begriffe, viele Fragen, wenig befriedigende Antworten

Was haben „evidenz-basierte" und „patientenorientierte" Medizin miteinander zu tun? Bedingen sie sich gegenseitig? Oder schließen sie einander aus? Die Antwort verlangt zunächst eine Definition der beiden Begriffe:

– Was ist *„patientenorientierte Medizin"*? Ist nicht jede Medizin patientenorientiert? Ohne Patienten gibt es keine Medizin!
– Was sollen wir unter *„Evidenz"* verstehen? Ist Evidenz eine Eigenschaft, die man einer richtigen Hypothese ansehen kann? Wenn wir das nicht können, wie beweisen Hypothesen ihre Richtigkeit?

4.1.1 Patientenorientierung

Patientenorientierung zu definieren, scheint auf den ersten Blick nicht schwierig zu sein. Viktor von Weizsäcker (1987) hat sie als eine Medizin definiert, die den Patienten als Subjekt in die Medizin einführt. Hier beginnen aber die Schwierigkeiten: Ist nicht jeder Patient ein Subjekt? Wie konnte die Medizin ihm diese Eigenschaft rauben? Und wenn sie es konnte, hat sie ihm diese Eigenschaft wiedergegeben und wenn ja, wie hat sie das gemacht? Man sollte glauben, dass diese Fragen zufriedenstellend beantwortet sind. Sie sind es aber nicht!

4.1.2 Evidenz und Evidenz-Basierung

Was ist nun aber Evidenz? Jetzt wird es wirklich schwierig: Das Philosophische Wörterbuch definiert Evidenz als die zentrale – wenn auch umstrittene – Instanz der offenkundigen, unmittelbar einleuchtenden Selbstbezeugung wahrer Erkenntnis (vgl. Ritter, 1972). Etwas einfacher ist es, wenn Evidenz etwas mit Erfahrung zu tun hat und dass es zwei verschiedene Definitionen für diese „Erfahrung" gibt, denen verschiedene Antworten auf die Frage entsprechen, was wir unter „Evidenz" verstehen.

4.2 Das wirkliche Anliegen der neuen Bewegung

D. L. Sackett (1997), einer der Pioniere der Bewegung, definiert evidenzbasierte Medizin als „Integration individueller klinischer Erfahrung mit der bestmöglichen externen Evidenz aus systematischer Forschung" bzw. „der gewissenhafte, ausdrückliche und vernünftige Gebrauch der gegenwärtig besten externen, wissenschaftlichen Evidenz für Entscheidungen über die medizinische Versorgung individueller Patienten" (vgl. Sackett et al., 1996). Das klingt einleuchtend und überzeugend, solange man die beiden Aspekte der Medizin, die hier integriert werden sollen, nicht genauer anschaut.

Der eine Aspekt, die „klinische Erfahrung" oder „interne Evidenz" wird als „das Können und die Urteilskraft definiert, die Ärzte durch ihre Erfahrung und klinische Praxis erwerben". Der andere, als „externe Evidenz" definierte Aspekt, besteht im Idealfall aus randomisierten kontrollierten klinischen Studien und systematischen Übersichten dieser Studien, die als „Goldstandard" bezeichnet werden, „da sie korrekt über die Frage informieren..., ob Therapiemaßnahmen mehr nützen als schaden".

Um diese externe Evidenz (EBM) für sich realisieren zu können, müsste ein Allgemeinarzt jeden Tag 19 Artikel aus nationalen und internationalen Zeitschriften lesen, und zwar an allen 365 Tagen im Jahr (vgl. Davidoff et al., 1995). Auch wenn das Internet oder das inzwischen gegründete Deutsche Cochrane Zentrum in Freiburg die Recherchezeit verkürzen, bleibt der zeitliche Aufwand für Fort- und Weiterbildung sehr hoch, um eine evidenz-basierte, abgesicherte therapeutische Entscheidung zu treffen. Weil es fast unmöglich ist, jede therapeutische Maßnahme entsprechend abzusichern, wundert es auch nicht, dass nur jede fünfte medizinische Maßnahme wissenschaftlich fundiert ist. Besonders wissenschaftsentrückt sind die Chirurgen: Etwa 94% der chirurgischen Vorgehensweisen sind nicht evidenz-basiert, entsprechen nicht einem standardisierten, regelhaften Vorgehen! Ist Chirurgie eine Kunst, ein Handwerk oder eine Wissenschaft?

„Interne Evidenz" steht also für das Wissen, das der praktisch tätige Arzt auf der Basis seiner täglichen Erfahrungen im Umgang mit Patienten in ihren individuellen Wirklichkeiten gewinnt, von denen jede ihre somatischen, psychischen und sozialen Probleme hat. Zur Gewinnung *externer Evidenz* werden diese individuellen Probleme durch randomisierte doppelblinde Verfahren eliminiert. So stellen beispielsweise multimorbide, vor allem ältere Patienten eine Kontraindikation für randomisierte, doppelblinde Studien dar. Komplexe diagnostische Probleme wie Wirbelsäulenbeschwerden, chronische Abdominalbeschwerden, das „chronique fatigue-Syndrom" oder die „chronische Prostatitis" werden in medizinischen Lehrbüchern nicht einmal erwähnt, weil weder Konzepte noch ein „Goldstandard" für diagnostische Standardverfahren existieren (vgl. Knottnerus und Dinant, 1997). Die angestrebte „Integration" interner und externer Evidenz heißt daher Elimination der internen Anteile und d. h. „Überwindung der subjektiven Urteile von Patienten und Ärzten" (vgl. FAZ, 31.12.97).

4.3 Der „Goldstandard" ist inflationär: Widersprüche von EBM

Die EBM-Bewegung hat aber leider eine falsche Geldwert-Philosophie: Der Goldstandard, der den Kurs-Wert einer Methode garantieren soll, hängt von der Wertschätzung ab, den die Methode genießt.

Unter dem Titel: „Die Macht der nicht-spezifischen Effekte des Heilens" erschien 1993 eine Arbeit (vgl. Roberts, 1993), in der eine chirurgische und vier internistische Therapiemethoden ausgewertet wurden, die seinerzeit aufgrund ihrer evidenten Wirksamkeit zu den wissenschaftlich anerkannten Verfahren, d. h. zum Goldstandard der Medizin gehörten[1]. Die Autoren werteten die Ergebnisse von 6.931 Fällen aus, die mit diesen Methoden behandelt wurden. Sie waren in der Tat eindrucksvoll: bei einem Drittel der Fälle ausgezeichnet, bei einem weiteren Drittel gut und nur bei einem Drittel nicht befriedigend. Leider konnten spätere Kontrollen die Erfolge nicht mehr reproduzieren, und die Methoden gerieten in Vergessenheit. Mit der Evidenz war die Effektivität der Verfahren geschwunden.

Die Autoren stellen die These auf, dass therapeutische Erfolge Ausdruck einer Konstellation sind, in der sowohl der Arzt als auch der Patient von der Wirksamkeit der Behandlung überzeugt sind. Da diese Konstellation bei jeder ärztlichen Behandlung eine Rolle spielt, muss man darüber nachdenken, wie diese Erfolge zu erklären sind. Dem steht aber das Fehlen einer Theorie im Wege, die dazu in der Lage ist. Die Elimination der subjektiven Urteile und Erwartungen der Beteiligten durch statistische Verfahren ist kaum ein Weg, der dieses Defizit zu beseitigen verspricht.

Die Liste der Beispiele für Widersprüche einer EBM ist lang:

Beispiel 1
Nach Schölmerich, Becher und Wittig (1997) wird fast bei jedem Patienten, der in einer inneren Abteilung einer Klinik stationär aufgenommen wird, eine Ultraschalluntersuchung und bei jedem zweiten Patienten eine com-

---

[1] Das chirurgische Verfahren bestand in der Entfernung des Glomus caroticum bei schwerem Asthma bronchiale, drei internistische Verfahren galten der Behandlung des Herpes simplex, das vierte war die Vereisung der Magenwand bei therapieresistenten Ulzera.

putertomographische Untersuchung durchgeführt. Trotzdem konnte durch die bildgebenden Verfahren die Anzahl der Fehldiagnosen in den letzten 20 Jahren nur von 78% auf 64% gesenkt werden, gleichzeitig hat sich die Zahl der pro Patient angewandten Verfahren verdoppelt, die Kosten sind sogar um das Sechsfache gestiegen. Die Fehldiagnosen konnten durch die Obduktionsbefunde gesichert werden, insbesondere konnte die Treffsicherheit bei pathologischen Abdominalbefunden durch eine größere Zahl von Tests nicht verbessert werden, insbesondere nicht bei lebensgefährlichen Erkrankungen der Nieren oder des Pankreas.

Beispiel 2
Bei Patienten mit schwerer Herzinsuffizienz wird die Substanz Milrinon, das die Kontraktilität des Myokards verbessert, eingesetzt. In der sogenannten PROMISE-Studie (Prospective Randomized Milrinone Survival Evaluation) wurden 1088 Patienten mit schwerer Herzinsuffizienz über 6 Monate mit Milrinon behandelt (vgl. Packer et al., 1991): Zu einer Senkung der Mortalität unter Milrinon kam es nicht, im Gegenteil: In der Verumgruppe lag die Mortalität bei 30%, in der Placebogruppe aber nur bei 24,1% (mit $p = 0.038$ statistisch signifikant).

Beispiel 3
Mit Encainid und Flecainid können ventrikuläre Arrhythmien nach einem Myocardinfarkt signifikant gegenüber Placebo gesenkt werden. Daraus könnte der Schluss gezogen werden, dass diese Antiarrhythmika das Risiko für einen plötzlichen Herztod senken. Nach der CAST-Studie (Cardiac Arrhythmia Suppression Trial) ist das Gegenteil der Fall: Bei insgesamt 730 über 10 Monate mit diesen Antiarrhythmika behandelten Herzinfarkt-Patienten betrug die Mortalität 7,7%, bei den insgesamt 725 mit Placebo behandelten Patienten der Vergleichsgruppe lag die Mortalität bei nur 3,3% (mit $p = 0.0003$ statistisch hoch signifikant) (vgl. CAST-Investigators, 1989).

4.4 Was ist Evidenz?

Die Hoffnung, durch ein philosophisches Lexikon zu erfahren, was eigentlich unter dem Zauberwort „Evidenz" zu verstehen ist, wird enttäuscht. Der Begriff ist seit seinem Auftauchen in der Antike umstritten. Statt dessen finden wir eine wichtige Spur: Evidenz hat mit „Erfahrung" zu tun, und da es verschiedene Definitionen für Erfahrung gibt, gibt es verschiedene Antworten auf die Frage, was unter „Evidenz" zu verstehen ist.

Die Definition der EBM-Bewegung, die randomisierte, doppelblinde Studien als „Goldstandard" bezeichnet, beruht auf dem empiristischen Erfahrungsbegriff, der auf John Locke (1632–1704) zurückgeht. Nach ihm muss sich ein Beobachter, der zuverlässige Erfahrungen machen will, in ein weißes Blatt Papier verwandeln, auf dem sich die beobachteten Sachverhalte unverfälscht abbilden können². Für den Arzt heißt das: Er muss seine subjektiven Gefühle, Vorstellungen zurücknehmen und durch die „objektiven Sachverhalte" randomisierter Studien ersetzen.

Eine Definition für „Evidenz", welche die Erfahrungen des Klinikers ernst nimmt, setzt einen anderen Erfahrungsbegriff voraus. Für ihn ist der Beobachter kein „weißes Blatt", sondern durch seine Fragestellung und Antwortmöglichkeiten geprägt, nach denen sich die Sachverhalte, die Erfahrung werden sollen, richten müssen. Dieser „Evidenz-Begriff" geht von der Definition für Erfahrung aus, mit der Kant 1784 die „konstruktivistische Wende" eingeleitet hat.

„Bisher nahm man an, alle unsere Erkenntnis müsse sich nach den Gegenständen richten – in den Worten Lockes wie ein unbeschriebenes Papier verhalten – (...). Man versuche es daher einmal, ob wir nicht (...) damit besser fortkommen, dass wir annehmen, die Gegenstände müssten sich nach unserem Erkennen richten (...)"

I. Kant „Kritik der reinen Vernunft" (1784, zit. n. Glasersfeld, 1996)

4.5 Pragmatische und kommunikative Evidenz

Evidenz-basierte Medizin will dem Arzt, so können wir ihr Anliegen positiv formulieren, eine ständige Fortbildung vermitteln, die ihm die Probleme seiner Patienten so darstellt, wie sie für den Arzt an der vordersten Linie der Forschung aussehen. Sie darf aber den Aspekt nicht ignorieren, den die Probleme für den Patienten – und in der Kommunikation zwischen Patient und Arzt – und d. h. für den Behandlungsauftrag haben. Hier begegnen wir dem anderen Evidenzbegriff und stehen immer wieder vor unvereinbaren Widersprüchen.

Heinz von Foerster (1993) hat auf dieses zentrale Problem der modernen Medizin eine Antwort gegeben. Sie geht davon aus, dass lebende Systeme „beobachtende Systeme" sind. Darunter versteht er Systeme, die ihre Umgebung unter dem Aspekt der Bedeutung erfahren, welche die Umgebung für sie hat. Er hat dann ein Modell entworfen, das beschreibt, wie lebende Systeme ihre Umgebung nicht als weiße Blätter erleben, sondern wie sie ihre Umgebung aufgrund der individuellen Formen ihrer Erfahrung, die durch ihre Bedürfnisse und Triebe geprägt sind, in die zu ihnen passenden Umwelten verwandeln. Oder kürzer formuliert: wie ihre Wahrnehmung ihre

---

[2] Für Locke stammen alle Begriffe und Erkenntnisse aus der Wahrnehmung, die für ihn mit Erfahrung identisch ist. In seinem Essay *„Concerning Human Understanding"* heißt es: *„all the materials of reason and knowledge"* kommen einfach in *„one word from experience"*, die mit *„perception"* gleichgesetzt wird. *„Let us than suppose the mind to be, as we say, white paper, void of all characters, without any ideas."*

Umgebung für ihre Probleme „in Form" bringt. Sie verhalten sich nach v. Foerster wie „logische Maschinen", die Veränderungen ihrer Rezeptoren als „Input" verwenden, den sie nach der Regel oder dem Sollwert eines Operators in einen „Output", die von ihnen wahrgenommene Umwelt, verwandeln.

Für unser Problem ist wichtig, dass v. Foerster zwei Typen solcher logischen Maschinen beschreibt: Eine Maschine, die jeden Input in einen technisch manipulierbaren Output verwandelt. Diesen Typus nennt er „triviale Maschine", weil ihr Operator jeden Input nach der Regel der mechanischen Kausalität in eine mechanische Ursache und jeden Output in eine mechanische Wirkung verwandelt. Sie trivialisiert ihre Umgebung, indem sie auf den gleichen Input unwandelbar mit dem gleichen Output antwortet. Diese logische Maschine ist für den Arzt der Prototyp, um Probleme eines Patienten in technisch manipulierbare Vorgänge zu übersetzen. Sie zeigt ihm die Probleme eines Patienten, wie sie für seine technischen Interventionsmöglichkeiten aussehen. Anders formuliert: Sie bringt die Probleme des Patienten für seine Eingriffe in Form, indem sie sie – und das kann lebensrettend sein – trivialisiert. Diese Maschine gehorcht einem „pragmatischen Realitätsprinzip", wie es in randomisierten Studien zum Ausdruck kommt. Sie produziert *pragmatische Evidenz*.

Das andere Modell ist die „nicht-triviale Maschine". Sie verwandelt, wie ihre triviale Schwester, jeden Input in einen Output. Aber ihr Operator arbeitet nicht nach der Regel der mechanischen Kausalität, sondern nach der wechselnden Bedeutung, die der Input für die Bedürfnisse des lebenden Systems hat, die sich mit jedem Arbeitsgang ändert. Die Maschine antwortet daher auf den gleichen Input mit einem anderen, dem ihrem inneren Zustand entsprechenden Output. Dieser Typus der logischen Maschine kann dem Arzt helfen, die Probleme zu sehen, wie der Patient sie wahrnimmt. Das ist die Voraussetzung, um sich mit ihm auf den Behandlungsauftrag zu einigen, der auch darin bestehen kann, sich vorübergehend für einen technischen Eingriff in Form zu bringen, d. h. trivialisieren zu lassen.

Die nicht-triviale Maschine folgt nicht einem „pragmatischen", sondern einem „kommunikativen Realitätsprinzip". Sie hilft dem Arzt, den Code zu erfassen, nach dem ein Kranker seine Wirklichkeit erlebt. Sie produziert keine pragmatische, sondern *kommunikative Evidenz*. Sie ist der wirkliche „Goldstandard", der Auskunft gibt, ob und inwieweit etwas, das der Arzt dem Patienten aufgrund pragmatischer Evidenz vorschlagen kann, unter dem Aspekt der kommunikativen Evidenz zwischen Arzt und Patient zu dem Patienten und seiner individuellen Situation „passt".

4.6 Die wissenschaftstheoretische Situation im 20. Jahrhundert

Zum Abschluss soll der Versuch unternommen werden, die Konsequenzen dieser Überlegungen auf dem Hintergrund der wissenschaftstheoretischen Situation im 20. Jahrhundert zu umreißen: In ihm haben sich – von der wissenschaftlichen Öffentlichkeit kaum zur Kenntnis genommen – die Einsichten Kants (vgl. Abschn. 4.4) bewahrheitet, dass sich die Gegenstände nach unserer Erkenntnis richten. Das war in der Quantenphysik die Konsequenz der Entdeckung des Beobachter-Problems bei Nils Bohr oder Werner Heisenberg (vgl. Bohr, 1935; Heisenberg, 1958), in der Biologie die Konsequenz der Umweltlehre, dargestellt von Jakob von Uexküll (vgl. v. Uexküll, 1936), und in der Psychologie die Konsequenz der Widerlegung der Abbildungstheorie bei Jean Piaget (vgl. Piaget,1967).

Seitdem müssen wir Wissenschaft neu definieren. Sie kann nicht mehr als das Bemühen verstanden werden, die Realität „hinter" unseren Beobachtungen aufzudecken. Die neue Definition ist bescheidener. Sie versteht Wissenschaft als Anstrengung, Zusammenhänge aufgrund definierter Ordnungsprinzipien herzustellen und zu erproben.

Für die Geschichte dieser Ordnungsprinzipien hat sich der Historiker Carlo Ginzburg (1983) interessiert und festgestellt, dass zwei Wissenschaftsformen existieren, die er „Indizienwissenschaften" und „galileische Wissenschaften" nennt. Die galileischen Wissenschaften haben unter der Führung der Physik in den letzten drei Jahrhunderten so weitgehend die Vorherrschaft errungen, dass Wissenschaft mit Physik gleichgesetzt wurde – und z. T. immer noch wird. Er kommt dann aber zu dem Ergebnis, dass nicht nur die Geschichtswissenschaften und die Jurisprudenz, sondern auch die Medizin Indizienwissenschaften sind, weil in ihnen das individuelle Moment entscheidend ist. Damit gerät sie mit den galileischen Wissenschaften in Konflikt, deren Forschungsmethoden die Mathematik und das Experiment sind.

Ginzburg schreibt dann:
„Der Gebrauch der Mathematik und die experimentelle Methode implizieren... die Wiederholbarkeit der Dinge – während eine individualisierende Wissenschaftsrichtung die Wiederholbarkeit per Definition ausschloss und die Quantifizierung nur als Hilfsfunktion zuließ..."

„Nun fällt die Gruppe der Wissenschaften, die wir – die Medizin eingeschlossen – Indizienwissenschaften nennen, keineswegs unter die Kriterien von Wissenschaftlichkeit, die das galileische Paradigma enthält. Es sind vielmehr im höchsten Grade qualitative Wissenschaften, die das Individuelle an Fällen, Situationen und Dokumenten zum Gegenstand haben, und die gerade deshalb zu Ergebnissen kommen, die einen Rest von Unsicherheit nie ganz vermeiden können." (S. 73)

„An diesem Punkt, heißt es dann, eröffnen sich nun zwei Möglichkeiten: Entweder man opfert die Erkenntnis des individuellen Elementes zu Gunsten der (mehr oder weniger streng mathematisch formulierbaren) Verallgemeinerung, oder man versucht – sich langsam vortastend – ein anderes Paradigma zu erarbeiten, das sich auf die wissenschaftliche Erkenntnis des Individuellen stützt (wobei es sich um eine Wissenschaftlichkeit handelt, die völlig neu zu definieren wäre). Den ersten Weg (auf dem man das individuelle Moment opfert) schlugen die Naturwissenschaften ein und, erst sehr viel später, die sogenannten Humanwissenschaften. Der Grund dafür ist offensichtlich: Die Tendenz, die individuellen Aspekte abzuwerten, ist direkt proportional zur emotionalen Distanz des Beobachters." (S. 79)

Wenn die Medizin die Tatsache zur Kenntnis nimmt, dass die Physik aufgehört hat, Leitwissenschaft der Naturwissenschaften zu sein, wie F. Cramer (1997), der Leiter des Max-Planck-Instituts für experimentelle Medizin in Göttingen[3], betont, muss sie sich auf sich selbst besinnen und „langsam zu einem anderen Paradigma vortasten".

---

[3] F. Cramer (S. 37): „In den letzten Jahren haben sich – von der wissenschaftlichen Öffentlichkeit meist unbemerkt – einige grundlegende Paradigmawechsel vollzogen, die damit zusammenhängen, dass die Physik als Leitwissenschaft der Naturwissenschaften allmählich abgelöst wird durch Biologie und Medizin."

4 Evidence-based and patient-oriented medicine: two models and how they are connected

Jörg Michael Herrmann, Glottertal
Thure von Uexküll, Freiburg

4.1 Preliminary note: two terms, many questions and few satisfactory answers

What is the connection between "evidence-based" and "patient-oriented" medicine? Is each conditional on the other? Or do they preclude each other? To answer these questions, the two terms must first be defined.

- What is *"patient-oriented medicine"*? Is not every kind of medicine patient-oriented? Without patients, there can be no medicine!
- What are we to understand by *"evidence"*? Is evidence a manifest property of a correct hypothesis? If it is not manifest, how do hypotheses prove that they are correct?

4.1.1 Orientation towards the patient

At first sight, it does not seem difficult to define patient orientation. According to the definition of Viktor von Weizsäcker (1987), patient-oriented medicine is a medicine in which the patient is introduced as a subject. However, this is where the difficulties begin. After all, is not every patient a subject? How was medicine able to rob him of this quality? And if it did manage to do so, has it given it back to him, and if so, how? One might imagine that these questions had been answered satisfactorily. Yet it turns out that they have not!

4.1.2 Evidence and evidence basing

But what actually is evidence? This is where things really do get difficult. Ritter's philosophical dictionary defines the German word "Evidenz" as the central – albeit disputed – agency of the manifest, immediately obvious self-attestation of true knowledge (cf. Ritter, 1972). Matters become rather simpler if evidence has something to do with experience and there are two different definitions of this "experience", each corresponding to different answers to the question of what we understand by "evidence".

4.2 The true intent of the new movement

D. L. Sackett (1997), one of the movement's pioneers, defines evidence-based medicine as the integration of "individual clinical expertise with the best available external clinical evidence from systematic research"; alternatively, it is "the conscientious, explicit and judicious use of current best evidence in making decisions about the care of individual patients" (cf. Sackett et al., 1996). This sounds self-evident and convincing until we take a closer look at the two aspects of medicine that are intended to be integrated here.

One of these aspects, "clinical experience" or "internal evidence", is defined as the "proficiency and judgment that individual clinicians acquire through clinical experience and clinical practice". The other aspect, defined as "external evidence", ideally consists of randomized controlled clinical studies and systematic reviews of these studies, which are described as a "gold standard for judging whether a treatment does more good than harm".

In order to procure this external evidence (EBM) for himself, a general practitioner would have to read 19 articles from national and international journals every day, 365 days a year (cf. Davidoff et al., 1995). Even if the Internet or the recently established German Cochrane Centre in Freiburg makes searching faster, the time required for continuing and post graduate education is substantial if an evidence-based therapeutic decision of confirmed validity is to be made. Since it is virtually impossible to confirm the validity of every therapeutic measure in this way, it is not surprising that only one medical measure in five is scientifically based. Surgeons are particularly remote from science: some 94% of surgical procedures are not evidence-based and do not correspond to a standardized method for which appropriate rules have been laid down! Is surgery an art, a craft or a science?

"Internal evidence" thus stands for the knowledge acquired by a practitioner on the basis of his day-to-day experience of and with patients in their individual realities, allowing for the fact that each patient has his or her own somatic, psychic and social problems. To obtain *"external evidence"*, these individual problems are eliminated by randomized double-blind techniques. For example, multimorbid patients – particularly older subjects – constitute a contraindication for randomized double-blind studies. Complex diagnostic problems such as disorders of the vertebral column, chronic abdominal pathology, "chronic fatigue syndrome" or "chronic prostatitis" are not even mentioned in medical textbooks, because neither concepts nor a "gold standard" exist for standard diagnostic procedures (cf. Knottnerus et al., 1997). Hence the aimed-for "integration" of internal and external evidence signifies elimination of the internal aspects – that is, "overcoming of the subjective judg-

ments of patients and doctors" (cf. Frankfurter Allgemeine Zeitung, 31 December 1997).

4.3 The "gold standard" is inflationary: contradictions of EBM

However, the EBM movement's philosophy of monetary value is unfortunately wrong: the gold standard that is supposed to guarantee the "market valuation" of a method depends on the esteem in which the method is held.

Some years ago, Roberts (1993) published a paper entitled "The power of nonspecific effects in healing", which contained an evaluation of one surgical and four internal-medicine treatments deemed at the time, owing to their manifest efficacy, to be scientifically recognized – i.e. treatments that belonged to the gold standard of medicine[1]. The authors evaluated the results of 6931 cases treated by these methods. The results were indeed impressive: excellent in a third of the cases, good in another third, and unsatisfactory in only a third. Unfortunately, the successes could not be reproduced in subsequent controls, and the methods were forgotten. The effectiveness of the procedures had disappeared with the evidence.

The authors postulate that therapeutic success is the expression of a constellation in which both the doctor and the patient are convinced of the efficacy of the treatment. Since this constellation plays a part in every medical treatment, it is important to reflect on the reasons for such successes. However, an obstacle to this reflection is the absence of a theory whereby this might be possible. Elimination of the subjective judgments and expectations of those concerned using statistical techniques is hardly an approach that promises to overcome this shortcoming.

The list of examples of contradictions in an EBM is long.

Example 1
According to Schölmerich et al. (1997), almost every in-patient in a clinic's medical ward undergoes an ultrasound examination and every other patient an examination by computer tomography. Even so, during the last 20 years the imaging techniques were able to reduce the number of misdiagnoses only from 78% to 64%; at the same time the number of procedures applied per patient doubled and costs increased by as much as a factor of six. The misdiagnoses were confirmed by autopsy findings; in particular, accuracy in the case of abdominal pathology could not be improved by increasing the

---

[1] The surgical procedure comprised removal of the carotid body in severe bronchial asthma; three of the internal-medicine methods were directed towards the treatment of herpes simplex; and the fourth was freezing of the stomach wall in patients with therapy-resistant ulcers.

number of tests, especially in non-life-threatening disorders of the kidneys or pancreas.

Example 2
The substance milrinone, which enhances the contractility of the myocardium, is used in patients with severe cardiac insufficiency. Under the "PROMISE" (Prospective Randomized Milrinone Survival Evaluation) study, 1088 patients with severe cardiac insufficiency were treated for six months with milrinone (cf. Packer et al., 1991). Rather than mortality being reduced by milrinone, the converse was found to be the case: mortality in the verum group was 30%, compared with only 24.1% in the placebo group (a statistically significant result at $p = 0.038$).

Example 3
Ventricular arrhythmias after myocardial infarction can be significantly reduced with encainide and flecainide as compared with placebo administration. This might lead one to conclude that these antiarrhythmics reduce the risk of sudden cardiac death. According to the CAST study (Cardiac Arrhythmia Suppression Trial), the opposite is the case: mortality in a total of 730 cardiac infarction patients treated with these antiarrhythmic agents over 10 months was 7.7%, compared with only 3.3% in the total of 725 placebo-treated patients in the control group (highly statistically significant, $p = 0.0003$) (cf. CAST Investigators, 1989).

4.4 What is evidence?

Our hopes of learning from a philosophical dictionary what the magic word "evidence" actually means prove to be disappointed. The term has been surrounded by controversy ever since it was first coined in antiquity. Instead, we find an important clue: evidence has to do with "experience", and since there are various definitions of experience, there are also a variety of answers to the question of what is to be understood by "evidence".

The definition of the EBM movement, which takes randomized double-blind studies as its "gold standard", is based on the empiricist notion of experience due originally to John Locke (1632–1704). In his view, an observer wishing to have reliable experience must turn himself into a white sheet of paper, upon which the observed situations can be reproduced without falsification[2]. For a physician, this means that he must abandon his subjective

---

[2] For Locke, all notions and knowledge are derived from perception, which he regards as identical with experience. He writes in his *Essay Concerning Human Understanding* that "all the materials of reason and knowledge" come simply in "one word from experience", which is equated with "perception": "Let us then suppose the mind to be, as we say, white paper, void of all characters, without any ideas."

feelings and ideas and replace them by the "objective situations" revealed by randomized studies.

A definition of "evidence" that takes the clinician's experience seriously demands a different notion of experience. For the clinician, the observer is not a sheet of "white paper", but is influenced by the question with which he is concerned and the possible answers to it, and the situations that are to become experience must accord with these. This "notion of evidence" derives from the definition of experience whereby Kant ushered in the "new constructivist era" in 1784:

"It has hitherto been assumed that all our cognition must conform to the objects – in the words of Locke, must behave like a blank sheet of paper – [...]. We should therefore consider whether we might not [...] make better progress by assuming that objects must conform to our cognizing ..."
 I. Kant "The Critique of Pure Reason" (1784, quoted in Glasersfeld, 1996)

4.5 Pragmatic and communicative evidence

The intent of evidence-based medicine can be formulated positively by saying that it sets out to provide the physician with a form of constant continuing education that presents his patients' problems to him in the way that they appear to a doctor at the forefront of research. However, it must not ignore the way the problems appear to the patient – and in the patient-doctor communication – and hence their relevance to the treatment contract. We here encounter the other notion of evidence and are confronted again and again with irreconcilable contradictions.

Heinz von Foerster (1993) suggested a solution to this central problem of modern medicine. It is based on the idea that living systems are "observing systems". By this he means systems that experience their environment in terms of the meaning it has for them. On this basis, he designed a model that describes how living systems do not experience their environment as white sheets of paper but instead transform it in accordance with the individual forms of their experience, as determined by their needs and drives, into one that suits them – in other words, how their perception shapes their environment in conformity with their problems. According to von Foerster, they behave like "logical machines" that use the changes in their receptors as "input", which they convert in accordance with the rule or reference value of an operator into an "output", namely the environment perceived by them.

The important point for our purposes is that von Foerster describes two types of logical machines. The first converts every input into a technically manipulable output. He calls this type a "trivial machine", because its operator, by the rule of mechanical causality, converts every input into a mechanical cause and every output into a mechanical effect. It trivializes its environment by responding to the same input immutably with the same output. For the physician, this logical machine is the prototype for translating a patient's problems into technically manipulable processes. It shows him a patient's problems in terms of his available stock of technical interventions. In other words, it shapes the patient's problems to suit his interventions by trivializing them – something that may be life-saving. This machine obeys a "pragmatic reality principle" as manifested in randomized studies. It produces *"pragmatic evidence"*.

The other model is the "non-trivial machine". Like its trivial counterpart, it converts every input into an output. However, its operator's rule is not mechanical causality but the changing significance of the input for the needs of the living system – a significance that alters with each action. The machine thus responds to one and the same input with a different output, corresponding to its internal state. This type of logical machine can help the doctor to see the problems as the patient perceives them. That is the condition for reaching agreement with the patient on the treatment contract, which may also consist in temporarily "shaping" him for a technical intervention – i.e., allowing himself to be trivialized.

The non-trivial machine obeys not a "pragmatic" but a "communicative reality principle". It helps the doctor to discern the code whereby a patient experiences his reality. It produces not pragmatic but *"communicative evidence"*. It is the true "gold standard", providing information as to whether, and to what extent, something the doctor can suggest to the patient on the basis of pragmatic evidence "fits" the patient and his individual situation from the point of view of the communicative evidence between doctor and patient.

4.6 The epistemological situation in the twentieth century

In conclusion, it shall be attempted to outline the consequences of these reflections against the background of the epistemological situation of the twentieth century. During this century, Kant's insight (cf. Section 4.4) that objects conform to our cognition – an insight barely noticed by the scientific public – proved accurate. This was a consequence, in quantum physics, of the discovery of the problem of the observer by Niels Bohr or Werner Heisenberg (cf. Bohr, 1935; Heisenberg, 1958); in biology, of Jakob von Uexküll's environmental theory (cf. von Uexküll, 1936); and in psychology, of Jean Piaget's refutation of the "copy theory" (cf. Piaget, 1967).

These realizations have necessitated a new definition of science. It can no longer be understood as the endeavour to discover the reality "behind" our observations. The new definition is more modest. It regards science as an effort to arrive at and test connections and correlations on the basis of defined principles of ordering.

4.6 The epistemological situation in the twentieth century

The historian Carlo Ginzburg (1983) investigated the history of these ordering principles and found that there are two forms of science, which he calls "sciences based on circumstantial evidence" and "Galilean sciences" respectively. The Galilean sciences enjoyed such hegemony under the leadership of physics in the last three centuries that science was – and to some extent still is – equated with physics. However, Ginzburg concludes that if the historical sciences and jurisprudence are sciences based on circumstantial evidence, so too is medicine, because the individual factor is decisive in all of them. Medicine thus comes into conflict with the Galilean sciences, whose methods of research are mathematics and experimentation.

Ginzburg continues: *"The use of mathematics and the experimental method imply [...] the reproducibility of things – whereas an individualizing scientific orientation by definition precluded reproducibility and allowed quantification only as an auxiliary function ..."*

"Now the group of disciplines – including medicine – which we call the sciences based on circumstantial evidence do not at all conform to the criteria of science contained in the Galilean paradigm. Rather, they are in the highest degree qualitative sciences, whose subject is the individual aspect of cases, situations and documents, and which, precisely for that reason, yield results that can never entirely avoid a residue of uncertainty" (p. 73).

"At this point, it is then asserted, there are two possibilities: either a knowledge of the individual element is sacrificed in favour of generalization (which can be formulated in more or less strictly mathematical terms), or an attempt is made, by feeling one's way slowly forward, to arrive at a different paradigm, based on scientific knowledge of the individual aspect (this being a kind of science calling for a completely new definition). The first approach (involving sacrifice of the individual factor) was opted for by the natural sciences and, only very much later, by the so-called human sciences. The reason is obvious: the tendency to devalue the individual aspects is directly proportional to the emotional distance of the observer" (p. 79).

If medicine takes note that physics has ceased to be the "master" natural science, as F. Cramer (1997)[3], the head of the Max Planck Institute of Experimental Medicine at Göttingen, has emphasized, it must undertake some self-reflection and "slowly feel its way towards a different paradigm".

---

[3] F. Cramer (p. 37): "In the last few years, mostly unnoticed by the scientific public, there have been some fundamental changes of paradigm, connected with the fact that physics has gradually been ousted from its position as the 'master' natural science by biology and medicine."

4.7 Literatur/References

Bohr, N.: Quantum Mechanics and Physical Reality. Nature, 136 (1935)

CAST-Investigators: Preliminary report. Effect of encainide and flecainide on mortality in a randomized trial of arrhythmia suppression after myocardial infarction. NEJM 321 (1989), 406–412

Cramer, F.: Gesundheit, Energie, Resonanz – ein Konzept der lebendigen Wechselwirkungen. In: Bartsch, H. H.; Bengel, J. (Hrsg.): Salutogenese in der Onkologie. Basel 1997, 37

Davidoff, F., Haynes, B., Sackett, D., Smith, R.: Evidence-based medicine: a new journal to help doctors identify the information they need. Brit med J 310 (1995), 1085–1086

FAZ: Eine Reformbewegung für die Kranken: Mehr Wissenschaft durch Evidenz-basierte Medizin/Überwindung subjektiver Urteile. FAZ vom 31.12.97

Foerster, H. v.: Wissen und Gewissen. Frankfurt 1993

Ginzburg, C.: Spurensicherungen. Berlin 1983

Glasersfeld, E. v.: Radikaler Konstruktivismus. Frankfurt 1996

Heisenberg, W.: Physics and Philosophy. The Revolution in Modern Science. New York 1958

Knottnerus, J. A., Dinant, G. J.: Medicine based evidence, a prerequisite for evidence-based medicine. Future research methods must find ways of accommodating clinical reality, not ignoring it. Brit med J 315 (1997), 1109–1110

Packer, M., Carver, J. R., Rodeheffer, R. J., Ivanhoe, R. J., Di Bianco, R., Zeldis, S. M., Hendrix, G. H., Bommer, W. J., Elkayam, U., Kukin, M. L., Mallis, G. J., Sollano, J. A., Shannon, J., Tandon, P. K., De Mets, D. L.: Effect of oral Milrinone on mortality in severe chronic heart failure. NEJM 325 (1991), 1468–1508

Piaget, J.: Six Psychological Studies. New York 1967

Ritter, J.: Historisches Wörterbuch der Philosophie, Band 2. Stuttgart 1972

Roberts, A. H.: The power of nonspecific effects in healing: Implications for psychosocial and biological treatments. Clinical Psychology Rev 13 (1993), 375–391

Sackett, D. L., Rosenberg, W. M. C., Gray, J. A. M., Haynes, R. B., Richardson, W. S.: Evidence based medicine: What it is and what it isn't. Brit med J 312 (1996), 71–72

Sackett, D. L. et al.: Was ist Evidenz-basierte Medizin und was nicht? Münch Med Wochenschr 139 (1997), 644–645

Schölmerich, J., Becher, H., Witzig, W.: Einfluß bildgebender Verfahren auf die prämortale Diagnosesicherheit. Med Klin 92 (1997), 394–400

Uexküll, J. v.: Umwelt als Insel und Ocean des Unerkennbaren. Was heißt Umwelt? In: Nie geschaute Welten. Fischer. Berlin 1936

Weizsäcker, V. v.: Ärztliche Fragen. Vorlesungen über Allgemeine Therapie. Gesammelte Schriften, Band 5. Frankfurt a. M. 1987

5 Evidenz-basierte Medizin und die Systematik der klinischen Entscheidungsfindung

Winfried Walther, Karlsruhe

5.1 Einleitung

Therapeutische Entscheidungen zu treffen, gehört zur Alltagsroutine des Zahnarztes. Dennoch ist kaum untersucht, auf welche Art und Weise über die Behandlung des individuellen Patienten entschieden wird und welche Faktoren die Entscheidung begründen. Zumeist tut der Zahnarzt „was funktioniert", ohne sich selbst darüber Rechenschaft zu geben, welche Beweggründe sein Handeln im Einzelfall bestimmen. Der Patient wiederum hält zumeist den Arzt für den Handelnden, der Entscheidungen für ihn und über ihn trifft. Selten nimmt er wahr, dass er selbst aktiv am Entscheidungsprozess teilnimmt. Die Komplexität und Dynamik der Therapiefindung wird deswegen weithin unterschätzt.

Die Darstellung eines Behandlungsfalles mit vielschichtigen Bewertungs- und Entscheidungsproblemen (vgl. Abb. 5-1) kann dies verdeutlichen. Die Patientin vertraut dem Zahnarzt, schildert ihr Leiden und hofft, durch den zahnärztlichen Eingriff hiervon befreit zu werden. Dem Zahnarzt fällt die Aufgabe zu, fachlich vertretbare Therapiealternativen zu entwickeln. Er entwirft diese Alternativen auf der Basis seines zahnmedizinischen Wissens. Hierfür sind zahlreiche Einzelentscheidungen zu treffen. Letztendlich kann jedoch nur eine der möglichen Behandlungsstrategien zur Anwendung kommen. Die Wahl dieser Strategie kann nicht allein aufgrund des angewandten normativen Wissens des Zahnarztes gefunden werden. Die Patientin wird die vorgestellten alternativen Behandlungswege vor dem Hintergrund ihrer Vorstellungen und der eigenen Interpretation ihres Leidens einschätzen und bewerten. Dies gilt prinzipiell auch bei Entscheidungsproblemen, die auf den ersten Blick einfacher strukturiert erscheinen als der hier dargestellte.

Da der klinische Entscheidungsprozess von den Beteiligten kaum reflektiert wird, löst der Begriff „evidenz-basierte Zahnheilkunde" sehr widersprüchliche Reaktionen aus. Auf der einen Seite wird befürchtet, mit ihm seien neue Vorschriften und Restriktionen verbunden, auf der anderen Seite wird erwartet, dass durch die mit ihm verbundene Verwendung der „besten externen wissenschaftlichen Evidenz für Entscheidungen in der medizinischen Versorgung" (vgl. Sackett, 1999) rationalere und zweckmäßigere Entscheidungen möglich

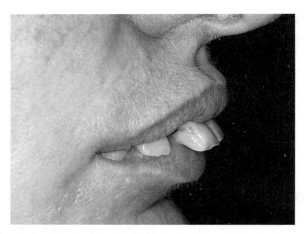

Abbildung 5-1: Behandlungsfall mit ästhetischer Problematik
Die Patientin leidet unter ihrem Erscheinungsbild und wünscht eine Verbesserung der ästhetisch unbefriedigenden Situation. Der Befund weist verschiedene tief greifende pathologische Veränderungen auf. Aus mehreren Therapiealternativen muss diejenige ausgewählt werden, die dem Anliegen der Patientin am ehesten gerecht wird und fachlicher Kritik standhält.

werden als bisher und dass die Zahnheilkunde dadurch besser und sicherer wird. Das Verstehen der klinischen Entscheidungsfindung ist somit der Schlüssel für die Frage, was durch evidenz-basierte Zahnheilkunde in Diagnostik und Therapie verändert wird und welche Auswirkungen auf das Arzt-Patienten-Verhältnis hierdurch zu erwarten sind.

Um Aufschluss über die Bedeutung des Konzeptes der „evidenz-basierten Zahnheilkunde" zu finden, sollen deswegen die folgenden Fragen untersucht werden:

– Welche Entscheidungsschritte sind Grundlage der systematischen Therapiefindung?
– Wie wird die Therapieentscheidung empirisch gesichert?
– Welche Bedeutung hat evidenz-basierte Zahnheilkunde für eine empirisch gesicherte Therapieentscheidung?
– Was sind die Merkmale der adäquaten Therapieentscheidung?

5.2 Welche Entscheidungsschritte sind Grundlage der systematischen Therapiefindung? Modelle der klinischen Entscheidungsfindung

Die Schritte der Therapiefindung lassen sich schematisch als Modell darstellen, wobei die wichtigen Entscheidungsgrundlagen benannt werden und

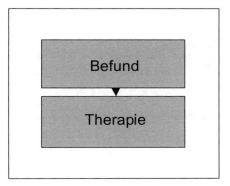

Abbildung 5-2: Modell Befund – Therapie

der Entscheidungsablauf veranschaulicht wird. Hierdurch kann deutlich gemacht werden, welche Konzepte der klinischen Entscheidungsfindung bestehen. Diese Konzepte bestimmen den Stellenwert, der der evidenz-basierten Zahnheilkunde zugewiesen werden muss.

Das einfachste Modell der klinischen Entscheidungsfindung wird in Abbildung 5-2 wiedergegeben (vgl. Abb. 5-2). Dieses Modell verdeutlicht den wichtigen Zusammenhang zwischen Therapie und vorausgehendem Befund. Ohne die Grundlage des klinischen Befundes ist die Therapieentscheidung undenkbar. Dieses Modell findet deswegen weithin Akzeptanz. Es muss jedoch festgestellt werden, dass es den realen Entscheidungsvorgang stark verkürzt. Es läuft auf die Konklusion hinaus, dass der Befund die Therapie determiniert, also nur eine Handlungsalternative zulässt. Komplexe Zusammenhänge zwischen Feststellungen und Folgerungen sind in diesem Modell nicht vorgesehen. Ferner kommen die Wirkung des Patientenwunsches und der Einfluss des zahnärztlichen Wissens als eigenständige Entscheidungsparameter nicht zum Ausdruck. Schlussfolgerungen, die auf Basis dieses Entscheidungsmodells getroffen werden, blenden somit wesentliche Bestandteile der klinischen Entscheidungsfindung aus.

Um diesem Defizit abzuhelfen, wird in Abbildung 5-3 ein Modell vorgestellt, in dem das Patientenanliegen und das angewendete zahnärztliche Wissen als entscheidungsrelevante Parameter eingeführt werden (vgl. Abb. 5-3).

Das Entscheidungswissen des Zahnarztes wird nach einem Vorschlag von Heners als „Therapeutische Software" bezeichnet (vgl. Heners, 2000; Heners und Walther, 2000). Dieser Begriff fasst den wissensgesteuerten Planungsprozess zusammen. Die tradierte Trennung zwischen Diagnose und Therapie wird in diesem Modell nicht aufgegriffen, da im ärztlichen Bereich kein kategorialer Unterschied zwischen „Erkennen" und „Handeln" besteht und häufig nicht „endgültige", sondern „Situationsdiagnosen" die Grundlage ärztlichen Handelns darstellen (vgl. Mannebach, 1997).

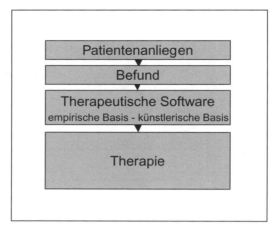

Abbildung 5-3: Entscheidungsmodell „Patientenanliegen – Befund – Therapeutische Software"

Das Entscheidungswissen des Zahnarztes umfasst nicht allein das während der zahnmedizinischen Ausbildung erworbene normative Wissen, sondern auch Erfahrungswissen, das der individuelle Behandler im Laufe seiner praktischen Tätigkeit erwirbt. Die Gesamtheit dieses Wissens wird als empirische Basis bezeichnet.

Der Zahnarzt wendet jedoch auch Wissen an, das eher einer künstlerischen als einer normativ-empirischen Basis zugerechnet werden kann. Vor allen Dingen bei ästhetisch wirksamen Eingriffen muss er versuchen, seine Arbeitsmittel und den Patientenwunsch optimal in Einklang zu bringen. Hierzu gehören Handlungsschritte, die eher intuitiv als rational gefunden werden und dennoch das Erscheinungsbild des Patienten nachhaltig beeinflussen. Die künstlerische Basis ist somit ein integrativer Bestandteil der „therapeutischen Software" des Zahnarztes, die im individuellen Entscheidungsfall große Bedeutung erlangen kann. Das klinische Entscheidungswissen hat somit unterschiedliche Ursprünge und bedarf deswegen einer differenzierten Betrachtung.

Das in Abbildung 5-3 vorgestellte Entscheidungsmodell führt zwar das Patientenanliegen als entscheidungsrelevanten Parameter ein, es sieht jedoch keine aktive Beteiligung des Patienten bei der Wahl der adäquaten Therapiealternative vor. Moderne Entscheidungstheorien der Therapiefindung gehen jedoch davon aus, dass dem Patienten eine sehr entscheidende Rolle bei dieser Wahl zufällt. Dies wird im nächsten Entscheidungsmodell ausgedrückt, das in Abbildung 5-4 vorgestellt wird und als „patientenorientiertes Entscheidungsmodell" bezeichnet werden soll (vgl. Abb. 5-4). Hier wird zwischen der Aufgabe des Arztes und der des Patienten unterschieden. Der Arzt formuliert auf Basis der Anamnese und des Befundes sowie unter Anwendung der „therapeutischen Software" fachlich begründete The-

5.2 Welche Entscheidungsschritte sind Grundlage der systematischen Therapiefindung? 107

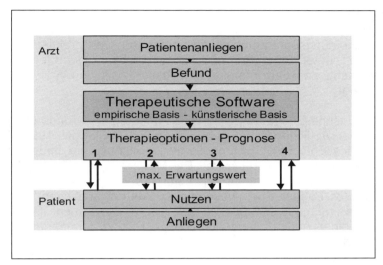

Abbildung 5-4: Patientenorientiertes Entscheidungsmodell: Der Zahnarzt konzipiert auf der Basis der „therapeutischen Software" Therapieoptionen, denen der Patient seinen subjektiv bestimmten Nutzen zuordnet. Die Therapieoption mit dem höchsten Erwartungswert ist die zu favorisierende.

rapiealternativen. Diese Therapiealternativen werden dem Patienten mitgeteilt. Als wesentliche Informationen sind Umfang und Art des Eingriffes sowie die verfügbaren Daten über seine Prognose zu betrachten. Der Patient wird so in die Lage versetzt, den Nutzen der einzelnen Therapiealternativen zu bestimmen.

Als letzter Schritt der Entscheidungsfindung steht in den Konzepten moderner Entscheidungstheorien die Maximierung des Erwartungswertes (vgl. Gross und Löffler, 1997; Koslowski, 1991). Der Erwartungswert ist das Produkt aus der Eintrittswahrscheinlichkeit des angestrebten klinischen Erfolges und dem erzielbaren Nutzen einer Therapie.

Die Mitwirkung des Patienten in dieser Entscheidungsphase ist von ausschlaggebender Bedeutung, da der Nutzen einer Therapie nicht aufgrund objektiver Parameter festgestellt werden kann, sondern der subjektiven Wertung des Patienten unterliegt (vgl. Gross und Löffler, 1997). Der Patient wird diese Wertung nicht nur auf sein Verständnis für die ihm erläuterten medizinischen Zusammenhänge gründen, sondern auch seine individuellen sozialen und psychologischen Bedingungen einbeziehen.

Die Therapieentscheidung stellt sich somit letztlich als Ergebnis eines kommunikativen Prozesses dar, der auf der „therapeutischen Software" und der Einschätzung des klinischen Problems durch den Patienten gründet. Diese komplexe Form der Entscheidungsfindung im Rahmen der Arzt-Patienten-Beziehung wird bei der Darstellung technisch-wissenschaftlich ausgerichteter Entscheidungsparameter häufig übersehen. Den praktisch-klinischen Bedingungen, unter denen Arzt und Zahnarzt arbeiten, wird jedoch nur ein Modell gerecht, das den interaktiven Prozess zwischen Arzt und Patient berücksichtigt.

Auch das ethische Gebot, den Willen des Patienten als Grundbedingung zur Ausübung der ärztlichen Kunst zu begreifen (vgl. Koslowski, 1991), kann im Rahmen eines Entscheidungsmodells nur dann Ausdruck finden, wenn es einen aktiven Patienten voraussetzt. Die Mitwirkung des Patienten bei der Therapiefindung gewinnt heute auch deswegen an Bedeutung, weil die Autonomie des Patienten als wesentliches Ziel der ärztlichen Tätigkeit erkannt wurde (vgl. v. Uexküll und Wesiak, 1998). Der Patient ist durch sein Leiden in seiner Autonomie beeinträchtigt. Richtig verstandene ärztliche Kunst fördert die Autonomie des Patienten, indem sie ihn durch den ärztlichen Eingriff zu selbstständigem Entscheiden und Handeln befähigt.

Die wesentlichen Entscheidungsparameter im patientenorientierten Entscheidungsmodell sind somit:

– Erhebung des Patientenanliegens (Anamnese),
– Befund,
– Einsatz der „therapeutischen Software" (empirische Basis und künstlerische Basis),
– Konzeption fachlich begründeter Behandlungsoptionen,
– Aufklärung über Behandlungsoptionen und deren Prognose,
– Erhebung des Nutzens für den Patienten,
– Suchen des höchsten Erwartungswertes.

Dieses Modell lässt erkennen, dass es nicht zweckmäßig ist, im individuellen Entscheidungsfall von einer richtigen bzw. falschen Entscheidung zu sprechen, da die Parameter fehlen, eine solche Wertung zu verifizieren. Angemessen ist vielmehr die Unterscheidung zwischen einer adäquaten und einer nicht adäquaten Entscheidung. Die adäquate Entscheidung wird getroffen unter Würdigung der medizinischen Voraussetzungen der Problemlösung sowie unter Einbeziehung der psychologischen und sozialen Bedingungen des Falles. Diese Bedingungen können nur durch die Mitwirkung des Patienten analysiert werden.

Durch das patientenorientierte Entscheidungsmodell kann auch abgeleitet werden, wie evidenz-basierte Zahnheilkunde in den Therapiefindungsprozess eingreift. Da die Verfahren der evidenz-basierten Zahnheilkunde auf eine Verbesserung der empirischen Wissensbasis des Zahnarztes abzielen, ist sie dem Bereich der „therapeutischen Software" zuzuordnen. Dies wird in Abbildung 5-5 veranschaulicht (vgl. Abb. 5-5). Evidenz-basierte Zahnheilkunde wird somit nicht zu einer völligen Neukonzeption der klinischen Pla-

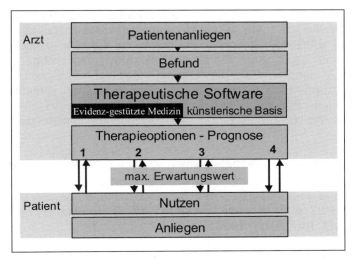

Abbildung 5-5: Die evidenz-basierte Zahnmedizin ist im Rahmen des patientenorientierten Entscheidungsmodells der empirischen Wissensbasis des Arztes zuzuordnen.

nung führen. Sie bewirkt eine Neuorientierung des Arztes im Bereich seiner empirischen Wissensbasis. Es kann keinesfalls erwartet werden, dass durch evidenz-basierte Methoden klinische Entscheidungsprobleme dergestalt aufgearbeitet werden, dass für einen individuellen Patienten eine „optimale" Therapieoption mit „maximaler Rationalität" bestimmt werden kann.

5.3 Wie wird die Therapieentscheidung empirisch gesichert?

Die „therapeutische Software" des Zahnarztes wird im Wesentlichen durch die zahnmedizinische Ausbildung geformt und im Laufe seiner praktischen Tätigkeit durch Erfahrung und Fortbildung ergänzt. Das Ausbildungssystem vermittelt Wissen mittels eines Trainingssystems, das durch traditionelle Lehrinhalte sowie durch Ergebnisse der Forschung bestimmt wird (vgl. Heners, 1991). Die Begründung des zahnärztlichen Eingriffs ist nicht in jedem Fall aus wissenschaftlichen Erkenntnissen ableitbar. Vielmehr kann unterschieden werden zwischen Entscheidungen auf Grundlage von:

– Konvention,
– Folgerungen aus Analogmodellen,
– Sicherheit und
– empirisch-stochastischen Begründungen.

Die Konvention, also die ungeprüfte Anwendung tradierter Regeln, bestimmt nach wie vor weite Teile der zahnmedizinischen Therapie. Schlussfolgerungen auf Grundlage von Experimenten in vitro (Analogschlüsse) sind ebenfalls hinsichtlich ihrer klinischen Bewährung nicht abgesichert, werden jedoch in der Regel als Begründung eines zahnärztlichen Eingriffs akzeptiert. Sicherheit als Entscheidungsgrundlage ist bei klinischen Problemen prinzipiell nicht gegeben, da die Zukunft eines klinischen Verlaufes unsicher ist und von den Bedingungen des individuellen Behandlungsfalles abhängt.

Deswegen wird heute als Begründung ärztlicher Maßnahmen die Anwendung von Ergebnissen aus der klinischen Forschung gefordert. Die wissenschaftliche Methode der Wahl ist hierbei die empirisch-stochastische Prüfung. Dies kommt in einer Forderung des Biometrikers Trampisch zum Ausdruck (vgl. Trampisch, 1993):

„Die Anwendung eines Therapiemittels allein aufgrund der Tatsache, dass es zu einem Therapiekonzept passt, welches auf einem pathophysiologischen Modell einer Erkrankung basiert, wird in der Medizin nicht mehr akzeptiert. Das Problem (der Unsicherheit durch die Individualität des Patienten) lässt sich nur mit kontrollierten klinischen Prüfungen lösen, in denen Aussagen über Erfolgswahrscheinlichkeiten getroffen werden."

Die klinische Prüfung steht in der Medizin somit zwischen der Hypothese (vermuteter Zusammenhang zwischen einem ärztlichen Eingriff und dem klinischen Verlauf einer Erkrankung) und der Formulierung einer allgemeingültigen Regel. Klinische Forderungen, die allein aufgrund eines Experimentes in vitro bestimmt wurden, bedürfen noch der Bestätigung im klinischen Experiment.

Um Wirkung und Tragweite klinischer Forschung zu verstehen, ist es erforderlich, die methodischen Voraussetzungen klinischer Prüfungen zu kennen. Im klinischen Experiment werden standardisierte Bedingungen für die wissenschaftliche Beobachtung angestrebt, um allgemein gültige Aussagen zu erwirken. Die wichtigsten Parameter der wissenschaftlichen Beobachtung sind:

– definierte Therapie(n),
– definierte Studienpopulationen,
– prognostische Variablen (Befund),
– Zeitachse,
– Response und Therapieerfolg.

Als Response wird die beobachtete Wirkung der Therapie bezeichnet. Diese ist im Allgemeinen eine Zustandsänderung (z. B. von „krank" zu „gesund"). Als Response können gemessen und beschrieben werden:

5.3 Wie wird die Therapieentscheidung empirisch gesichert?

- organische Veränderungen,
- technische Veränderungen (z. B. am Zahnersatz) und
- subjektives Empfinden.

Die Definition der Response-Variablen erfordert immer eine Abstraktion des angestrebten Therapieerfolges, da die Therapiewirkung nicht nur für einen einzelnen Patienten festgelegt wird, sondern in einer Patientengruppe beobachtet werden soll. Somit muss ein eindeutig objektivierbarer Zustandswechsel gefunden und der Untersuchung zu Grunde gelegt werden.

Das Ergebnis der wissenschaftlichen Beobachtung drückt den Behandlungserfolg aus, indem es eine Aussage über die Responsevariable in Abhängigkeit von der verwandten Therapie und den prognostischen Variablen trifft.

Die Aussage kann vorliegen in Form einer:

- Häufigkeit,
- Wahrscheinlichkeit (Eintrittswahrscheinlichkeiten, Wahrscheinlichkeit von Zusammenhängen),
- Differenz von Häufigkeiten und/oder Wahrscheinlichkeiten.

Als Beispiel zeigt die Abbildung 5-6 zwei Überlebenskurven von Pfeilerzähnen nach Inkorporation eines prothetischen Ersatzes (vgl. Abb. 5-6). Die Abbildung lässt erkennen, dass der Vergleich von Therapien nie zu dem Er-

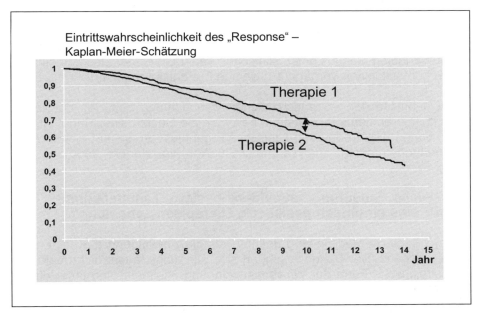

Abbildung 5-6: Überlebenskurven als Ergebnis einer klinischen Fragestellung zum Erfolg vergleichbarer Therapien

gebnis kommt, dass eine klinische Methode prinzipiell versagt, während die andere zum Erfolg führt. Vielmehr wird ein gradueller Unterschied gefunden, der jetzt mit den Methoden der Stochastik weiter untersucht werden kann. Es muss insbesondere die Frage geklärt werden, ob der Unterschied zufallsbedingt entstand oder durch die Therapie zu erklären ist.

Die Aussagen klinischer Studien werden an definierten Studienpopulationen erhoben, die meist in Versuchsgruppen aufgeteilt wurden. Diese Aufteilung wird nach Möglichkeit methodisch so ausgeführt, dass eine Verallgemeinerung des Ergebnisses möglich ist (randomisierte, also zufällige Zuteilung zu den Versuchsgruppen).

Die wissenschaftliche Beobachtung sichert:

– die Indikationsstellung bekannter Therapieverfahren und
– die Anwendung neuer Therapieverfahren.

Gerade bei der Einführung neuer Verfahren stellt das Ergebnis einer klinischen Prüfung den einzigen Maßstab dar, der es gestattet, die neue Methode mit bekannten Verfahren zu vergleichen und zu bewerten.

Die hier vorgestellte, abstrahierende Betrachtung von klinischen Studienergebnissen lässt erkennen, dass derartige Ergebnisse niemals direkt die Form einer klinischen Regel annehmen können. Der in der Prüfung dokumentierte Erfolg ist immer unter bestimmten Voraussetzungen zustande gekommen. Vor der Übernahme in eine Regel muss deswegen geprüft werden, ob in der Praxis entsprechende Bedingungen zutreffen oder einzuführen sind. Ferner drückt die Aussage über eine oder wenige isolierte Responsevariablen niemals einen klinischen Verlauf in seiner Gesamtheit aus, da sie den wirklichen Vorgang auf wenige Ereignisse reduziert.

Die Ergebnisse der wissenschaftlichen Beobachtung bedürfen deswegen einer fachgerechten Interpretation, bevor sie die Gestalt einer Regel annehmen können. Die Bedeutung klinischer Ergebnisse erschließt sich in ihrer unvoreingenommenen Analyse und Diskussion (vgl. Heners, 2000).

5.4 Welche Bedeutung hat evidenz-basierte Zahnheilkunde für eine empirisch gesicherte Therapieentscheidung?

Evidenz-basierte Medizin wird definiert als die Anwendung der besten externen Evidenz. Der Begriff erschöpft sich allerdings längst nicht mehr auf eine spezifische Form der Wissensanwendung. Vielmehr sind unter dieser Bezeichnung neue Methoden des Erwerbes, der Interpretation und auch der Wertung von Wissen vorgestellt und angewendet worden. Diese Verfahren werden von internationalen, wissenschaftlichen Netzwerken eingesetzt und stellen das eigentlich Neue an der evidenz-basierten Medizin dar.

5.4 Welche Bedeutung hat EBD für eine empirisch gesicherte Therapieentscheidung?

Evidenz-basierte Medizin kann als Update der „therapeutischen Software" verstanden werden, wobei zwei bedeutsame Qualitätsaspekte Berücksichtigung finden:

– die Anwendbarkeit im klinischen Entscheidungsprozess und
– die Verallgemeinerungsfähigkeit des wissenschaftlichen Outputs (Abwendung von Verzerrungen – Bias).

Für diesen Zweck sind wichtige Werkzeuge entwickelt worden. Die bedeutsamsten sind der „systematische Review" und die „kritische Bewertung" (critical appraisal). Der „systematische Review" umfasst die Sammlung und Auswertung vorhandener wissenschaftlicher Originalarbeiten, die nach festgelegten Regeln ausgeführt wird. Hierbei wird auf eine möglichst vollständige Erhebung des verfügbaren Wissens und auf eine standardisierte Gegenüberstellung der Ergebnisse geachtet. Die „kritische Bewertung" erfolgt, indem eine vorhandene Studie methodisch festgelegten Fragestellungen unterworfen wird (Beispiel siehe Tabelle 5-1). Diese Form der Untersuchung ermöglicht die Entscheidung der Frage, ob für die getroffene Aussage eine starke oder nur eine schwache Evidenz angenommen werden kann.

Die durch die evidenz-basierte Medizin eingeführten Methoden fußen alle auf der Auswertung von bereits verfügbarer wissenschaftlicher Literatur. Sie streben keine eigenständige Erhebung wissenschaftlicher Erkenntnisse an. Evidenz-basierte Medizin bezweckt vielmehr, entscheidungsrelevante wissenschaftliche Beobachtung auf systematische Weise

– zu sammeln,
– verfügbar zu machen,
– zusammenzuführen und zu vergleichen,
– zu werten (kommentieren) und
– die Ergebnisse zu kategorisieren und zu archivieren.

Tabelle 5-1: Methodische Fragestellung zur Untersuchung einer veröffentlichten Meta-Studie (Auszug; Methodik des NHS Centre for Reviews and Dissemination)

– Author's objective
– Specific interventions included in the review
– Participants included in the review
– Outcomes assessed in the review
– Criteria on which the validity (or quality) of studies was assessed
– How were the judgements of validity (or quality) made?
– How were the studies combined?
– Results of the review
– Author's conclusions
– CRD (Centre for Reviews and Dissemination) commentary

Evidenz-basierte Medizin beabsichtigt somit nicht die systematische Erhebung von entscheidungsrelevanten wissenschaftlichen Daten. Sie gibt auch keine systematischen Problemlösungsstrategien für den individuellen Entscheidungsfall vor. Neben den direkt bezweckten Wirkungen wird sie jedoch sicher zu einer immer stärkeren Standardisierung der klinischen Forschung führen. Ferner ist zu erwarten, dass durch sie die wissenschaftliche Begründung klinischer Entscheidungen ständig an Bedeutung gewinnt. Angesichts der Tatsache, dass vielfach noch Konvention und Folgerungen aus Analogmodellen die Grundlagen zahnärztlicher Regeln bilden, ist zu hoffen, dass evidenz-basierte Zahnheilkunde die wissenschaftliche Grundlage der Zahnheilkunde stärken und der kritischen Diskussion über die Wirkung zahnärztlicher Eingriffe eine neue Qualität verleihen wird.

Diese sich nun einstellende Diskussion wirft jedoch Fragen auf, die bei der Erörterung klinischer Probleme nicht aus den Augen gelassen werden dürfen. So ist zu klären, wer die strukturierte, unvoreingenommene Diskussion über den wissenschaftlichen „Update" verantworten soll. Der Zahnarzt sollte nicht passiv die Ergebnisse einer solchen Diskussion entgegennehmen, sondern aktiv an ihr beteiligt sein. Angesichts vielfältiger Bestrebungen, im Rahmen der evidenz-basierten Zahnheilkunde auch Leitlinien zu formulieren, erhebt sich die Frage, ob diese Leitlinien als autoritäre Feststellung auf unbekannter Wissensbasis angestrebt werden oder durch eine strukturierte Diskussion über offen gelegte Erkenntnisse erarbeitet werden sollen. Und auch hier stellt sich die Frage, wer die Interpretationshoheit über vorgelegte wissenschaftliche Ergebnisse hat – einige wenige Experten oder jeder, der fachlich begründete Entscheidungen treffen muss?

Es ist zu erwarten, dass der Zahnarzt, will er in der Diskussion um klinische Begründungen standhalten, seine eigene Dokumentation den Erfordernissen dieser Diskussion anpassen muss. Es wird in Zukunft nicht mehr genügen, auf eigene klinische Erfahrung hinzuweisen. Die Erfahrung muss dokumentiert und nachprüfbar sein. Der Zahnarzt hat hierdurch die Chance, ein eigenes Gegengewicht zur externen Evidenz aufzubauen und selbst aktiv an den Grundlagen der Diskussion mitzuwirken (vgl. Heners und Walther, 2000; Walther, 1990, 1998).

5.5 Was sind die Merkmale der adäquaten Therapieentscheidung?

Die Akquisition von Wissen mit den Methoden der evidenz-basierten Medizin wird in Zukunft einen wesentlichen Beitrag dazu leisten, die Wirksamkeit ärztlicher und zahnärztlicher Eingriffe zu sichern. Dennoch ist nicht zu erwarten, dass sie externe Richtlinien begründen kann, die dem Arzt das Handeln im individuellen Entscheidungsfall vorschreiben. Arzt und Zahnarzt werden weiterhin gemeinsam mit dem Patienten um die adäquate Problemlösung des individuellen Entscheidungsfalles ringen. Die adäquate Entscheidung ist durch mehrere gleichwertige Parameter gekennzeichnet. Sie

- ist mit wissenschaftlichen Daten begründet,
- kunstvoll,
- getroffen auf der Basis des Patientenanliegens und der Würdigung der psycho-sozialen Bedingungen des Entscheidungsfalls,
- respektiert die Autonomie des Patienten und
- fördert sein Wohlergehen.

5 Evidence-based medicine and the systematics of clinical decision-making

Winfried Walther, Karlsruhe

5.1 Introduction

Making therapy decisions is a part of the dentist's everyday routine. However, hardly any research has been done on the way decisions are made on the treatment of an individual patient and on the factors that underlie these decisions. The dentist usually does "what works", without any attempt to justify to himself the motives that have determined his actions in a particular case. The patient, in turn, as a rule sees the practitioner as the active party who takes decisions for and about him. He seldom realizes that he himself plays an active part in the decision-making process. For this reason, the complexity and dynamics of the process of deciding on the appropriate therapy tend to be greatly underestimated.

This can be illustrated by the following clinical case, which presents a variety of different problems of assessment and decision-making (see Fig. 5-1). The patient trusts the dentist, describes her condition to him and hopes that it will be relieved through the dental intervention. The dentist is faced with the task of establishing therapeutic alternatives valid in terms of his specialty. He does this on the basis of his knowledge of dentistry. For this purpose, a large number of individual decisions must be made. Ultimately, however, only one of the possible treatment strategies can be implemented. The choice of this strategy cannot be made solely on the basis of the dentist's applied normative knowledge. The patient will appraise and assess the suggested alternative therapies against the background of her own ideas and interpretation of her condition. The same will be true of decision problems whose structure is at first sight simpler than that described here.

Since the protagonists devote little conscious thought to the process of clinical decision-making, the concept of "evidence-based dentistry" gives rise to very contradictory reactions. On the one hand people fear that it may involve new regulations and restrictions, but on the other there is an expectation that, because it calls for the use of the "best external scientific evidence for decisions in medical care" (cf. Sackett, 1999), it will allow more rational and more appropriate decisions than hitherto, so that dentistry will as a result become better and more certain. An understanding of the process of clinical

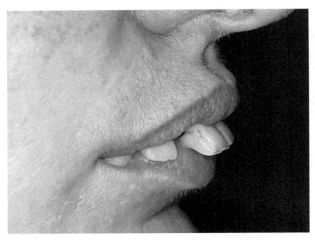

Figure 5-1: A clinical case involving aesthetic considerations
The patient is pained by her appearance and hopes for an improvement of the aesthetically unsatisfactory situation. Clinical examination reveals various severe pathological alterations. Several options for therapy suggest themselves and it is a matter of choosing the one that will best conform to the patient's wishes while at the same time standing up to professional criticism.

decision-making thus provides the key to identifying what is changed in diagnosis and therapy by evidence-based dentistry and what the likely effects on the doctor/dentist-patient relationship will be.

To provide some indication of the meaning of the concept of "evidence-based dentistry", the following questions will therefore be examined:

– What decision-making steps underlie systematic determination of the appropriate therapy?
– How is the decision on therapy underpinned empirically?
– What is the significance of evidence-based dentistry for an empirically underpinned therapeutic decision?
– What are the characteristics of appropriate decision-making on therapy?

5.2 What decision-making steps underlie systematic determination of the appropriate therapy? Models of clinical decision-making

The steps in determination of the appropriate therapy can be schematized in a model, in which the main elements underlying the decision are named and the process of decision-making is illustrated. In this way the specific concepts of clinical decision-making can be made explicit. These concepts determine the value to be assigned to evidence-based dentistry.

5.2 What decision-making steps underlie systematic determination of therapy?

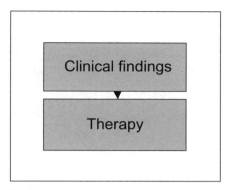

Figure 5-2: Findings-therapy model

The simplest model of clinical decision-making is illustrated in Figure 5-2 (see Fig. 5-2). This model shows the important connection between therapy and the prior clinical findings. A decision on therapy is inconceivable without the foundation of the clinical findings. This model is therefore widely accepted. However, it is manifestly a highly condensed representation of the actual process of decision-making. It suggests that the findings determine the therapy – i.e. that they admit of only one option for action. This model does not allow for complex connections between findings and conclusions. Furthermore, the effect of the patient's wishes and the influence of specialized dental knowledge do not feature as autonomous decision-making parameters. Conclusions based on this decision model thus exclude important constituents of the process of clinical decision-making.

To remedy this shortcoming, Figure 5-3 depicts a model in which the patient's wishes and the dental knowledge applied are introduced as parameters relevant to the decision process (see Fig. 5-3).

Heners suggests that the dentist's decision-making knowledge should be called "therapeutic software" (cf. Heners, 2000; Heners & Walther, 2000). This term embraces the whole of the knowledge-controlled planning process. The traditional separation of diagnosis and therapy is disregarded in this model, because there is no difference of category between "investigation" and "action" in the medical field and because medical action is frequently based not on "definitive diagnoses" but on "situation diagnoses" (cf. Mannebach, 1997).

The dentist's decision-making knowledge comprises not only the normative knowledge acquired during dental training but also the experience-based knowledge amassed by the individual practitioner during the course of his professional activity. The totality of this knowledge is described as the "empirical basis".

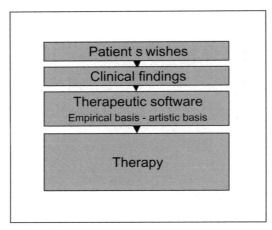

Figure 5-3: Decision model based on "patient's wishes–findings–therapeutic software"

However, the dentist also applies knowledge whose basis must be seen as artistic rather than normative and empirical. With interventions intended to have aesthetic effects in particular, he must seek optimum harmonization of his working instrumentarium with the patient's wishes. This will involve actions chosen on the basis more of intuition than of reason, although they will permanently affect the patient's appearance. The artistic basis is thus an integral part of the dentist's "therapeutic software", which may assume great importance in individual decision situations. Hence clinical decision-making knowledge has various origins and a number of different aspects must be considered.

Although the decision model presented in Figure 5-3 introduces the patient's wishes as a parameter relevant to the decision, it does not allow for active participation by the patient in the choice of the appropriate therapeutic option. However, modern theories on therapeutic decision-making assume that the patient plays a very decisive part in this choice. This is expressed in the next decision model, which is illustrated in Figure 5-4 and will be described as the "patient-oriented decision model" (see Fig. 5-4). It distinguishes between the task of the dentist and that of the patient. On the basis of the anamnesis and the clinical findings, as well as of his "therapeutic software", the dentist formulates therapeutic options in accordance with accepted professional practice. The patient is informed of these alternatives. The information will concern mainly the scale and nature of the intervention and the available data on the patient's prognosis. In this way the patient is enabled to determine the benefit of the individual therapeutic options.

The final step in the decision-making process, according to modern decision theories, is maximization of expected value (cf. Gross & Löffler, 1997;

5.2 What decision-making steps underlie systematic determination of therapy?

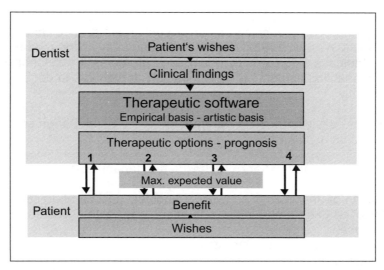

Figure 5-4: Patient-oriented decision model: On the basis of the "therapeutic software" the dentist devises options for therapy, to which the patient assigns his subjectively determined benefit. The therapeutic option with the highest expected value is the one to be favoured.

Koslowski, 1991). The expected value is the product of the probability of occurrence of the hoped-for clinical result and the achievable benefit of a therapy.

The patient's participation in this phase of decision-making is of crucial importance, as the benefit of a therapy cannot be determined on the basis of objective parameters but is a matter of the patient's subjective appraisal (cf. Gross & Löffler, 1997). This appraisal will not only be based on the patient's understanding of the medical considerations as explained to him, but also be influenced by his individual social and psychological reality.

The decision on the appropriate therapy thus ultimately is the outcome of a process of communication based on the "therapeutic software" and on the patient's assessment of the clinical problem. This complex form of decision-making in the context of the doctor/dentist-patient relationship is often overlooked in descriptions of decision-making parameters based on technical and scientific considerations. However, the practical and clinical conditions in which doctors and dentists work are fully allowed for only by a model that takes account of the interactive process between doctor/dentist and patient.

Again, the ethical precept that the will of the patient should be seen as the fundamental condition for the exercise of the medical art (cf. Koslowski, 1991) can be expressed only in a decision model that assumes an actively participating patient. Another reason for the increased importance now attached to patient participation in the choice of therapy is that the patient's autonomy has been recognized as an essential aim of medical activity (cf. von Uexküll & Wesiak, 1998). The patient's autonomy is impaired by his pathology. Medical art as correctly understood promotes the autonomy of the patient by enabling him, through the medical intervention, to decide and act independently.

The principal decision-making parameters in the patient-oriented decision model are thus as follows:

– determination of the patient's wishes/needs (anamnesis),
– clinical findings,
– application of "therapeutic software" (empirical basis and artistic basis),
– identification of treatment options in accordance with accepted professional practice,
– informing the patient about treatment options and their prognosis,
– identification of benefit to the patient,
– maximizing expected value.

This model indicates that a decision in an individual case cannot be described as right or wrong, because the parameters for verifying this judgment are lacking. What is more to the point is to distinguish between an appropriate and an inappropriate decision. An appropriate decision is taken with due regard for the medical preconditions for solving the problem at hand and at the same time for the psychological and social circumstances of the case. These circumstances can be analysed only with the patient's participation.

The patient-oriented decision model also indicates how evidence-based dentistry affects the process of determining the appropriate therapy. Since the methods of evidence-based dentistry are directed towards improving the dentist's empirical knowledge base, EBD must be assigned to the field of "therapeutic software". This is illustrated in Figure 5-5 (see Fig. 5-5). Evidence-based dentistry will thus not lead to a completely new conception of clinical planning, but has the effect of reorienting the dentist's empirical knowledge base. It is quite unrealistic to expect that, through evidence-based methods, problems of clinical decision-making will be transformed in such a way as to allow the determination of an "optimum" therapy option of "maximum rationality" for an individual patient.

5.3 How is the decision on therapy underpinned empirically?

The dentist's "therapeutic software" is substantially formed by his dental education and added to during the course of his professional activity by experience and continuing education. Dental training imparts knowledge by a system combining traditional syllabus content and research results (cf. He-

5.3 How is the decision on therapy underpinned empirically?

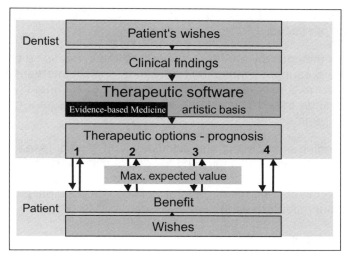

Figure 5-5: In the patient-oriented decision model, evidence-based dentistry must be assigned to the dentist's empirical knowledge base.

ners, 1991). The justification of a dental intervention cannot always be derived from scientific evidence. Decisions may instead be based variously on the following:

– convention,
– conclusions from analogy-based models,
– certainty, and
– empirical-stochastic verification.

Convention – i.e. the unverified application of traditional rules – continues to govern wide areas of dental therapy. Conclusions based on in vitro experiments (conclusions by analogy) are also not clinically proven, but are as a rule accepted as justification for a dental intervention. Certainty can never form the basis for decision-making in clinical problems, as a future clinical course of events is uncertain and depends on the conditions of the individual clinical case.

For this reason, the use of clinical research results is currently demanded as justification for medical measures. The scientific method of choice here is empirical-stochastic verification. This is expressed in the following demand by the biometrician H.-J. Trampisch (cf. Trampisch, 1993):

"The use of a means of therapy solely because it conforms to a therapeutic concept based on a pathophysiological disease model is no longer accepted in medicine. The problem [of uncertainty due to the patient's individua-

lity] can be solved only by controlled clinical trials yielding statements as to probabilities of success."

Clinical trials thus occupy an intermediate position in medicine between hypothesis (the presumed connection between a medical intervention and the clinical course of a disease) and the formulation of a generally valid rule. Clinical demands based solely on in vitro experiment require confirmation by clinical experiment.

An understanding of the effect and significance of clinical research calls for a knowledge of the methodological conditions of clinical trials. Standardized conditions for scientific observation are aimed for in clinical experimentation in order to permit statements of general validity. The principal parameters of scientific observation are as follows:

– defined therapy/therapies,
– defined study populations,
– prognostic variables (findings),
– time axis,
– response – result of therapy.

The observed effect of the therapy is called the "response". This is in general a change of state (e.g. from "sick" to "healthy"). The following responses can be measured and described:

– organic changes,
– technical changes (e.g. in dentures), and
– subjective experience.

Definition of the response variables always necessitates an abstraction of the aimed-for clinical result, since the therapeutic effect is not only specified for an individual patient but also supposed to be observed in a group of patients. This means that an unequivocally objectivizable change of state must be found and taken as the basis for the study.

The result of the scientific observation expresses the outcome of the treatment in the form of a statement about the response variable depending on the therapy used and of the prognostic variables.

This statement may take the following forms:

– frequency,
– probability (probabilities of occurrence or of correlations),
– differences between frequencies and/or probabilities.

As an example, Figure 5-6 shows two survival curves for abutment teeth after incorporation of a prosthesis (see Fig. 5-6). The diagram shows that a comparison of therapies never comes to the result that one clinical method

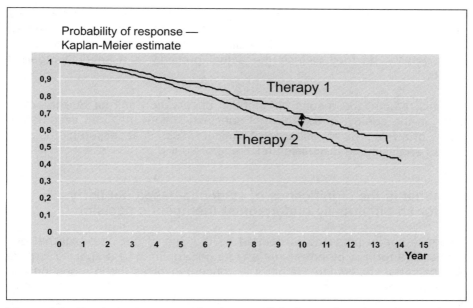

Figure 5-6: Survival curves resulting from a clinical question about the results of comparable therapies

always fails while another leads to success. What is found, rather, is a gradual difference, which can now be investigated further by stochastic methods. In particular, it must be ascertained whether the difference was due to chance or can be explained by the therapy.

The results of clinical studies are obtained from defined study populations, usually divided into experimental groups. Where possible, the methodology adopted for this division is chosen so as to allow generalization of the result (randomized – i.e. chance – apportionment among the experimental groups).

Scientific observation underpins:

- the indications for known therapeutic procedures, and
- the use of new therapeutic procedures.

Precisely when new procedures are introduced, the result of a clinical trial is the only criterion whereby the new method can be compared with known procedures and assessed.

The abstract consideration of clinical study results described here indicates that such results can never directly assume the form of a clinical rule. The result documented in a trial has always been obtained under specific conditions. Before it is transposed into a rule, it is therefore necessary to verify whether corresponding conditions apply or should be introduced in the practical situation. Again, results for a single response variable, or a small number of response variables, in isolation never express a clinical course in its totality, as they reduce the actual process to a small number of events.

For this reason, the results of scientific observation call for due interpretation in the context of the relevant speciality before they can assume the status of a rule. The significance of clinical results is assessed by their unbiased analysis and discussion (cf. Heners, 2000).

5.4 What is the significance of evidence-based dentistry for an empirically underpinned therapeutic decision?

Evidence-based medicine is defined as the use of the best external evidence. The term is by no means any longer confined to a specific form of application of knowledge. Rather, the concept involves the introduction and application of new methods of acquiring, interpreting and also rating knowledge. These methods are used by international scientific networks and constitute the truly new element in evidence-based medicine.

Evidence-based medicine can be regarded as an update of the "therapeutic software" in which two important aspects of quality are taken into account:

– applicability in the clinical decision-making process, and
– generalizability of the scientific output (avoiding distortion/bias).

Important tools have been developed for this purpose. Chief among these are systematic review and critical appraisal. "Systematic review" comprises the collection and evaluation of existing original scientific papers by predetermined rules. The aim here is as complete as possible recording of the available knowledge and standardized comparison of the results. "Critical appraisal" takes the form of subjecting an existing study to methodologically determined questions (see Table 5-1 for an example). This form of investigation makes it possible to decide whether strong or only weak evidence may be assumed in support of the stated result.

The methods introduced by evidence-based medicine are all based on the evaluation of already available scientific literature. They do not seek to establish new scientific knowledge independently. The purpose of evidence-based medicine is, instead, systematically

– to collect,
– to make available,
– to collate and compare, and

5.4 What is the significance of EBD for an empirically underpinned therapeutic decision? 127

– to appraise (comment on)
  scientific observations relevant to decision-making, and
– to categorize and archive the results.

Table 5-1: Methodological questions for examining a published meta-study (extract; methodology of the NHS Centre for Reviews and Dissemination)
– Author's objective – Specific interventions included in the review – Participants included in the review – Outcomes assessed in the review – Criteria on which the validity (or quality) of studies was assessed – How were the judgments of validity (or quality) made? – How were the studies combined? – Results of the review – Author's conclusions – CRD (Centre for Reviews and Dissemination) commentary

Evidence-based medicine is thus not concerned with the systematic establishment of scientific data relevant to decision-making. Nor does it offer systematic problem-solving strategies for individual decision-making situations. Apart from the directly intended effects, however, it will surely lead to the increasing standardization of clinical research. In addition, scientific justification of clinical decisions is likely to become more and more important as a result of EBM. Since many dental rules are still based on convention and on conclusions from analogy-based models, it may be hoped that EBD will reinforce the scientific foundations of dentistry and impart a new quality to the critical debate on the effects of dental interventions.

However, this nascent debate raises questions that must not be lost sight of in the discussion of clinical problems. For example, who is to be responsible for the structured, unbiased debate on the scientific "update"? The dentist should not passively accept the results of such a debate, but instead be an active participant in it. Efforts are also in hand to formulate guidelines in a number of spheres in the context of evidence-based dentistry, and the question therefore arises whether these guidelines should take the form of authoritarian statements on an unknown foundation of knowledge or be drawn up by way of a structured debate on disclosed findings. Here again, who will be deemed competent to interpret scientific results presented – a small number of experts, or anyone who has to make decisions required to be solidly underpinned within the relevant specialty?

If dentists wish to make valid contributions to the debate on clinical justification, they will presumably have to match their own documentation to the requirements of this debate. It will no longer suffice in future to point to one's own clinical experience. Experience must be documented and verifiable.

The dentist thus has an opportunity to build up countervailing material of his own to the external evidence and himself to take an active part in the fundamentals of the debate (cf. Heners & Walther, 2000; Walther, 1990, 1998).

5.5 What are the characteristics of appropriate decision-making on therapy?

The acquisition of knowledge by the methods of evidence-based medicine will in future make an important contribution to underpinning the effectiveness of medical and dental interventions. It is, however, unlikely to constitute an appropriate foundation for external directives prescribing how the doctor/dentist is to proceed in making an individual decision. Doctors and dentists will continue to struggle together with their patients to find the appropriate problem solution in an individual decision-making case. The appropriate decision is characterized by a number of parameters, each of which enjoys equal status. This decision will:

– be justified by scientific data,
– be artistic,
– be taken on the basis of the patient's wishes and allow for the psychosocial conditions relevant to the decision in the particular case,
– respect the patient's autonomy, and
– promote the patient's well-being.

5.6 Literatur/References

Gross, R., Löffler, M.: Prinzipien der Medizin – Eine Übersicht ihrer Grundlagen und Methoden. Heidelberg 1997

Heners, M.: Die Bedeutung allgemein anerkannter Regeln und ihrer Kriterien für die Qualitätsdiskussion in der Zahnmedizin. Dtsch Zahnärztl Z 46 (1991), 262–266

Heners, M.: Abschied vom Handwerkermodell Zahnheilkunde. Zahnärztl Mitt 90 (2000), 33–43

Heners, M., Walther, W.: Zahnärztliche Qualitätssicherung. Schweiz Monatsschr Zahnmed 110 (2000), 51–57

Koslowski, P.: Ärztliches Engagement und rationale Entscheidungsregeln. Zur Problematik ärztlichen Handelns innerhalb allgemein anerkannter Regeln. Dtsch Zahnärztl Z 46 (1991), 182–185

Mannebach, H.: Die Struktur des ärztlichen Denkens und Handelns. Weinheim 1997

Sackett, D. L.: Was ist Evidenz-Basierte Medizin? In: Perleth, M., Antes, G. (Hrsg.): Evidenzbasierte Medizin – Wissenschaft im Praxisalltag. München 1999

Trampisch, H.-J.: Stochastisches Denken als unverzichtbare Grundlage für wissenschaftliche Erkenntnis und praktisches Handeln in der Medizin. In: Köbberling, J.: Die Wissenschaft in der Medizin – Selbstverständnis und Stellenwert in der Gesellschaft. Stuttgart 1993

Uexküll von, T., Wesiak, W.: Theorie der Humanmedizin – Grundlagen ärztlichen Denkens. München 1998

Walther, W.: Kontinuierliche Beobachtung zahnärztlicher Behandlungsfälle durch subsequente EDV-gestützte Dokumentation. Dtsch Zahnärztl Z 45 (1990), 160–162

Walther, W.: Die subsequente Dokumentation der Zahnärztlichen Akademie – ein Informationssystem zur Sicherung der zahnärztlichen Therapieentscheidung. In: Dudek, D. (Hrsg.): Zahnärztl Welt – Spezial, Computer in Zahnarztpraxis und Dentallabor. Heidelberg, 1998

6 Evidenz-basierte Zahnheilkunde als Grundlage der prothetischen Therapie

Thomas Kerschbaum, Köln

6.1 Vorbemerkung

Klinische Entscheidungen in der zahnärztlichen Prothetik beruhen derzeit ganz überwiegend auf drei Faktoren: 1. der Erfahrung, die der einzelne Zahnarzt in seinem Beruf sammeln konnte bzw. auf die er sich durch Ausbildung und Kenntnis von Publikationen bezieht, 2. seinen Wertvorstellungen und Intuitionen sowie 3. den verfügbaren Ressourcen (vgl. Muir Gray, 1997). In dieser Trias spielt bisher die meinungsbasierte Entscheidung über die geeignete prothetische Therapie traditionell die wichtigste Rolle. Warum ähnliche Befunde im Kauorgan eines Patienten zu völlig unterschiedlichen Therapieansätzen bei enormen Kostenunterschieden führen können, kann durch diese Vorgehensweise erklärt werden. Zunehmender Druck auf die verfügbaren Ressourcen und die vermehrte Akzeptanz vergleichender wissenschaftlicher Therapiestudien zwingen jedoch dazu, evidenz-basierte Therapieentscheidungen in der Prothetik zu fördern und dadurch gleichzeitig auch Qualitätssicherung zu betreiben.

Es muss vor allem den praktischen Zahnarzt und die Studenten der Zahnmedizin irritieren, dass sie in ihrer Ausbildung mit zahlreichen „Gesetzen" und „Regeln" wie der anteschen Regel, dem thielemannschen Diagonalgesetz, der Hanau Quint, dem Costen-Syndrom, dem Károlyi-Effekt (vgl. Türp und Antes, 2000) vertraut gemacht wurden, ohne dass die Evidenz dieser Regeln wissenschaftlich begründet ist. Kritisch beurteilt wird der geringe Anteil gesicherten Wissens in der Zahnmedizin: Böning (2000) sprach von 8%, Marinello (1999) von 10–15%, ohne genau mitzuteilen, auf welcher Grundlage diese Schätzungen beruhen.

6.2 Warum evidenz-basierte Entscheidungen?

Es gibt derzeit vier wesentliche Gründe, sich Gedanken darüber zu machen, evidenz-basierte Leitlinien für die zahnärztliche Prothetik zu entwickeln und einzuführen (mod. nach Böning, 2000):

- Prothetische Maßnahmen haben eine wichtige Bedeutung für die Lebensqualität des Menschen.
- Zahnprothetik verursacht hohe Kosten im Gesundheitssystem.
- Es bestehen unangemessene Qualitäts- und Kostenunterschiede zwischen möglichen Versorgungsalternativen.
- Eine Verbesserung der Versorgungsqualität erscheint sinnvoll.

Zahnersatz bestimmt heute in einem beträchtlichen Ausmaß unsere Lebensqualität, wie aus den aktuellen bevölkerungsrepräsentativen Statistiken und Befragungen (vgl. Walter, Roediger und Rieger, 1999; Walter et al., 1999; IDZ, 1999) hervorgeht (vgl. Tab. 6-1). Kumuliert man alle prothetischen Therapiemaßnahmen von der Einzelkrone bis zur Totalprothese, so übersteigt Zahnersatz bereits in der Altersgruppe 35–44 Jahre die 50%-Grenze, d. h. ab dieser Altersgruppe nimmt bereits jeder zweite Einwohner derartige Therapieformen in Anspruch. In den höchsten Altersgruppen halten fast alle Menschen in Deutschland Zahnersatz für notwendig (vgl. Abb. 6-1) und messen ihm besondere Bedeutung für ihre Lebensqualität bei. Der Grund ist leicht nachvollziehbar: Trotz aller Erfolge und Bemühungen in der Prophylaxe gehen heute noch in Deutschland zwischen dem 35. und 64. Lebensjahr durchschnittlich 10–15 Zähne verloren. In der Altersgruppe 65–74 Jahre sind derzeit ein Viertel aller Einwohner in Deutschland zahnlos und tragen Vollprothesen. Gesellschaftliche Normen und andere Gründe (Ästhetik, Sprache, Kaufunktion) sorgen dafür, dass sich niemand dem „Zwang", Zahnersatz zu tragen, entziehen kann.

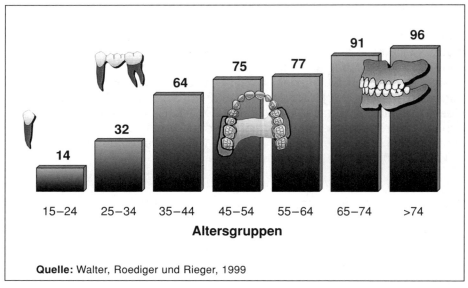

Quelle: Walter, Roediger und Rieger, 1999

Abbildung 6-1: Häufigkeit von Zahnersatz in Prozent

Tabelle 6-1: Zahnersatz in mittleren und höheren Altersstufen			
		35–44 Jahre	65–74 Jahre
		%	%
Teilprothese	OK	5,8	28,3
Teilprothese	UK	6,7	36,2
Totalprothese	OK	2,1	41,8
Totalprothese	UK	1,1	26,2
Totalprothese	OK/UK	1,1	24,0
Quelle: IDZ: DMS III, 1999			

Für Zahnersatz wurden nach neuesten Daten rd. 35% (nominal rd. 11 Mrd. DM) aller Kosten aufgewendet, die insgesamt in der Zahnmedizin 1996 eingesetzt wurden (rd. 35 Mrd. DM) (vgl. hochgerechnete Daten von Bauer, Neumann und Saekel, 1994). Zahnmedizinische Kosten sind heute zu einem erheblichen Teil an den Gesundheitskosten in Deutschland (pro Jahr rd. 550 Mrd. DM) beteiligt. Für Zahnersatz musste ein typischer Haushalt (West) nach Angaben des Statistischen Bundesamtes 1998 durchschnittlich 536 DM an Zuzahlungen im Jahr einplanen – mehr als für jeden anderen Sektor der Gesundheitsausgaben (z. B. Arzneimittel).

Über die Qualität der zahnärztlichen Versorgung, insbesondere über Zahnersatz, wurde immer wieder effekthaschend und meist negativ berichtet (vgl. z. B. Spiegel-Report über Qualitätsmängel in der zahnärztlichen Versorgung 12/1990; Studie „Markttransparenz beim Zahnersatz" des WIdO, Bauer und Huber, 1999). Neben aller berechtigten Kritik an derartigen Studien (vgl. Walther und Meyer, 1999), müssen aber auch Meinungsdifferenzen und -unsicherheiten über eine adäquate befundorientierte Therapie konstatiert werden. So ist beispielsweise die alltäglich vom Zahnarzt zu entscheidende Frage, ob ein Zahn noch mit einer plastischen (oder gegossenen) Füllung versorgt werden kann oder überkront werden muss, keineswegs geklärt (vgl. Covey et al., 1999; Staehle, 1999) oder auch nur durch hinreichend schlüssige Antworten abgedeckt. Die Frage, ob eine Krone oder Füllung erneuert werden muss oder belassen werden kann, lässt sich bisher nicht anhand klarer, nachvollziehbarer Kriterien entscheiden, obwohl Re-Dentistry heute vermutlich den größten Teil der Beträge, die für zahnmedizinische Zwecke ausgegeben werden, verschlingt. Die Liste alltäglicher zahnärztlicher Verrichtungen, die durch unterschiedliche Auffassungen gekennzeichnet sind, ließe sich fast unendlich verlängern. Dies gilt ganz spezifisch auch für typisch prothetische Probleme: Abbildung 6-2 zeigt die sechs Alternativen einer prothetischen Versorgung bei einem fehlenden Frontzahn (vgl. Abb. 6-2), Abbildung 6-3 listet die typischen Behandlungsalternativen im Freiendbereich auf (vgl. Abb. 6-3) und Tabelle 6-2 trägt Kosten und mittlere Überlebensraten zusammen (vgl. Tab. 6-2).

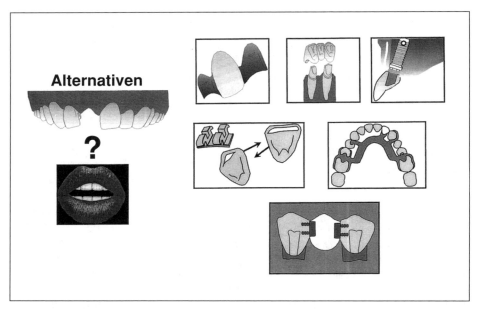

Abbildung 6-2: Behandlungsalternativen bei einer Frontzahnlücke (Adhäsivbrücke, konventionelle Brücke, Einzelimplantat, kieferorthopädischer Lückenschluss, partielle Prothese, UDA-Brücken [wegen erhöhter Kariesanfälligkeit im Ankerbereich nicht mehr indiziert])

Tabelle 6-2: Kosten und mittlere Überlebensdauer verschiedener prothetischer Therapiemittel		
Versorgung	Index Kosten	Survival in Jahren
Kunststoff-Prothese	0.2	3
Modellguss-Prothese	0.5	8
Adhäsivbrücke	0.5	10
Metallkeramik-Brücke	1.0	20
Einzelimplantat	1.6	20
Quelle: Öwall, Käyser und Carlsson, 1996, S. 14 (übersetzt)		

6.3 Quellen der Evidenz in der Prothetik

6.3.1 Internet

Schaut man in den typischen Internetquellen (NHS-Center for Reviews and Dissemination, The University of York, The Cochrane Collaboration, Center for Evidence-based Dentistry, Institute of Health, EBM/Ulm, AWMF-State-

6.3 Quellen der Evidenz in der Prothetik

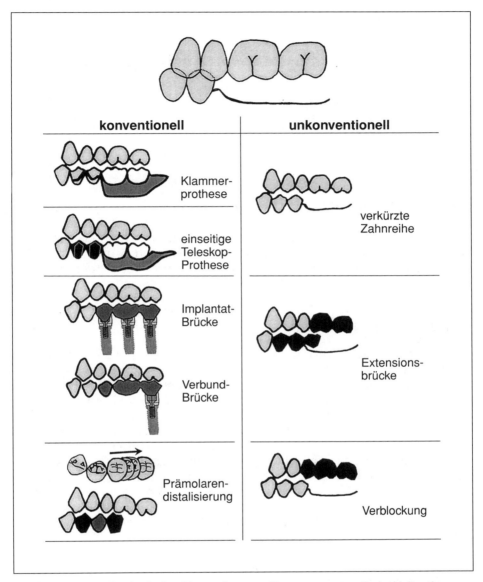

Abbildung 6-3: Prothetische Alternativen zur Versorgung von Freiendsituationen

ments, Health Evidence Bulletins/Wales, Stichwort: Oral health) nach, so findet sich dort sehr wenig Fachspezifisches unter dem Stichwort Zahnersatz. Kiefergelenkerkrankungen und orofaziales Schmerz-Syndrom werden behandelt (auch bei AWMF), extremer Zahnverschleiß wird thematisiert. Evidenz-basierte prothetische Leitlinien oder auch nur Ansätze wurden nicht entdeckt.

6.3.2 Meta-Analysen

Unter dem Begriff „Meta-Analyse" (Suchzeitraum: 1994 bis 1999) wurden in Medline 25 Treffer registriert, von denen nur vier prothetische Themen betrafen:

- Verblendschalen (Veneers),
- Überlebenszeiten von Brücken (2x),
- Adhäsiv-Brücken.

6.3.2.1 Veneers

Meijering (1997) und Kreulen, Creugers und Meijering (1998) werteten insgesamt 39 Studien über den Einsatz von Keramik- und Kunststoffschalen aus den Jahren 1983 bis 1996 aus und kamen zu dem Ergebnis, dass das Überleben von keramischen Veneers (n = 1552) nach 4 Jahren mit 92 % günstiger ausfiel, als wenn Kunststoffschalen verwendet wurden (n = 323), von denen nach 3 Jahren nur noch 78 % in Funktion standen.

6.3.2.2 Brücken

Langzeitstudien aus Kliniken und Praxen auf der Basis von systematisch geführten Karteien und Dokumentationen (zahnärztliche Behandlungsunterlagen, Versicherungsakten) gestatten eine nahezu lückenlose Übersicht über die Verweildauer, d. h. das Schicksal von Kronen und Brücken seit ihrer Eingliederung. Dabei werden heute nur noch zeitbezogene Aussagen (z. B. Kaplan-Meier-Kurven, vgl. Kaplan und Meier, 1958) akzeptiert. In den nachfolgenden Tabellen 6-3 und 6-4 werden zwei Meta-Analysen (vgl. Creugers, Käyser und van't Hof, 1994; Scurria, Bader und Shugars, 1998) gewürdigt, die sich mit der Überlebensrate von (festsitzenden) Brücken und ihren Pfeilern beschäftigt haben (vgl. Tab. 6-3 und 6-4). Nach diesen Ergebnissen haben zwei Drittel aller Brücken nach 15 Jahren unter Funktion ihre therapeutische Aufgabe noch erfüllt. Rund 96–98 % aller Pfeilerzähne waren nach 10 Jahren unter Therapie noch in Funktion.

6.3.2.3 Adhäsivbrücken

Hierzu gibt es mehrere Übersichten mit meta-analytischem Charakter: Creugers und van't Hof (1991) sowie Kerschbaum und Haastert (1995) stellten fest: Adhäsivbrücken sind vorzugsweise im kariesfreien und jugendlichen Gebiss bei kleinen, zahnbegrenzten Lücken indiziert. Sie sind komplikationsreich in der Nachsorge: Nahezu jede zweite Brücke löst sich mindestens einmal in 10 Jahren.

Tabelle 6-3: Langzeitergebnisse zum Überleben von Kronen und Brücken

Kronen				
Erstautor	Jahr	Anzahl	Zeit (Jahre)	Überlebens-rate (%)
Westermann	1990	222	8	88
Kerschbaum	1991	4371	15	59
Erpenstein	1992	593	15	84
BKK-Studie	1992	20946	6	94
Schlösser	1993	390	9	93
Langel	1994	112	8	89
Nordmeyer	1996	472	5	99
Stoll	1999	1679	10	86 *(Teilkr.)*
Brücken				
Erstautor	Jahr	Anzahl	Zeit (Jahre)	Überlebens-rate (%)
Leempoel	1987	1674	12	87
Kerschbaum	1991	1669	15	64
Erpenstein	1992	298	15	60
BKK-Studie	1992	2578	6	97
Creugers	1994	Meta-Analyse	15	74
Seth	1995	2583	10	76
Nordmeyer	1996	131	5	98
Scurria	1998	Meta-Analyse	15	75

Quelle: Kerschbaum, 2000

6.3.3 DGZMK-Statements

Den unregelmäßig erscheinenden Stellungnahmen der DGZMK kann in Deutschland durchaus Leitliniencharakter auf Expertenniveau zuerkannt werden. Von den insgesamt 88 aktuellen Statements (Stand: 12/99) betrafen aber nur 11 prothetische Themen (vgl. Tab. 6-5). Vergleicht man die DGZMK-Stellungnahmen mit leitlinienähnlichen Publikationen anderer Fachgesellschaften auf zahnmedizinischem Gebiet (z. B. AWMF), so muss man den DGZMK-Statements auf prothetischem Gebiet eine solide Aussagekraft und Kompetenz bescheinigen.

Tabelle 6-4: Langzeitergebnisse zum Überleben von Pfeilerzähnen

Erstautor	Jahr	Pfeiler Kronen/Brücken Anzahl	Zeit (Jahre)	Überlebensrate (%)
Hain	1993	222	8	96 *(Voll-/Teilkr.)*
Schlösser	1993	390	9	99 *(Vollkronen)*
Schlösser	1993	725	9	99 *(Teilkronen)*
Schlösser	1993	588	9	96 *(Brücken)*
Langel	1994	112	10	98 *(Kronen)*
Seth	1995	3313	10	96 *(Brücken)*
Scurria	1998	1525	10	96 *(Brücken (MK))*
Quelle: Kerschbaum, 2000				

Tabelle 6-5: Anzahl DGZMK-Statements in zahnmedizinischen Fachgebieten (Stand 12/99)

Themen	n
Allgemeines	31
Konservierende Zahnmedizin	17
Prothetik	11
Chirurgie	9
Parodontologie	6
Präventive Zahnmedizin	8
Kieferorthopädie	3
Röntgenologie	3
Gesamt	**88**

6.3.4 Ausländische Fachgesellschaften (USA)

Schon der Name „Parameters of Care" des American College of Prosthodontists (März 1996) signalisiert, dass das 70-seitige Papier als eine Art Leitlinie gedacht war. Es deckt konsequent alle Tätigkeitsfelder dieses Fachgebietes ab: Klinische Befunderhebung und -bewertung, Veränderungen am Einzelzahn, partielle und totale Zahnlosigkeit, Implantatprothetik, ästhetische Prothetik, Behandlung von Kiefergelenkpatienten, Epithetik und Resektionsprothetik, Behandlung von Schlafstörungen, Lokalanästhesie und adjuvante Maßnahmen. Vermittelt werden u. a. Standards, Richtlinien zur Indikation, therapeutische Ziele, Risikofaktoren. Schaut man genauer hin, so werden jedoch nur Kapitelüberschriften von Lehrbüchern zusammengetragen. Ihnen fehlen alle Merkmale, die EBD ausmachen. Ein Beispiel: Ob ein Zahn überkront werden muss oder noch gefüllt werden kann, wird auf die Schlagworte: Verlust von Zahnhartsubstanz und ihre Ursachen beschränkt (Karies, Attrition, Erosion, Abfraktion, Frakturen und Infraktionen, endodontische Therapie).

6.4 Problematik prothetischer Leitlinienentwicklung

6.4.1 Allgemeines

Für viele zahnmedizinische Tätigkeitsfelder gilt inzwischen, dass eine fast unüberschaubare Anzahl von Zeitschriften und Artikeln die analytische Arbeit erschwert: Jährlich erscheinen weltweit rd. 42 000 zahnmedizinische Artikel in rd. 490 Zeitschriften (vgl. Spiekermann, 1999). Eine Übersicht zu bestimmten Themen oder Fragestellungen ist daher nicht mehr ohne weiteres (Suchhilfen in medizinischen Datenbanken wie Medline) zu gewinnen.

Wichtiger als der quantitative Aspekt erscheint aber das Qualitätsproblem: Dumbrigue, Jones und Esquivel (1999a; 1999b) stellten bei einer Untersuchung der international wichtigsten drei prothetischen Journale (Journal of Prosthetic Dentistry, International Journal of Prosthodontic Dentistry, Journal of Prosthodontic Dentistry) fest, dass von den insgesamt 3 631 Artikeln nur 62 randomisierte, klinisch kontrollierte Studien (sog. RCTs) waren. Das bedeutet bestenfalls 1,7 % aller internationalen prothetischen Artikel erreichten das höchste Evidenzniveau. Schon Windeler stellte 1996 in einem Aufsatz enttäuscht fest, dass die Studien in den führenden Zeitschriften in Deutschland, wie der DZZ (41 %), und in den USA, Journal of Dental Research (20 %) und Journal Clinical Periodontology (75 %), patienten-orientiert waren. Ein weitaus geringerer Teil dieser Studien war nach den Regeln von „good clinical practice" (GCP) konzipiert.

In einem Fächervergleich von Badovinac, Conway und Niederman (1999) wurde belegt, dass in der Zahnmedizin signifikant weniger häufig RCTs (randomisierte, kontrollierte klinische Studien) und MAs (Meta-Analysen) erscheinen, verglichen mit kleineren medizinischen Fächern oder Disziplinen (Kardiologie, Gasteroenterologie, Infektiologie, Dermatologie, Muskel-/Skeletterkrankungen, Endokrinologie, Hämatologie).

Über die Gründe, warum in der Zahnmedizin, speziell in der Prothetik, ein derart beklagenswertes Niveau herrscht, spekulierte Böning (2000):

– *Die hohe Lehrbelastung bindet erhebliche Ressourcen; dazu kommen Patientenversorgung und organisatorische Probleme.*

– *Das Prinzip „publish or perish" bestimmt mehr und mehr die zahnmedizinische Forschungslandschaft; Langzeitstudien werden erst gar nicht durchgeführt, weil die Ergebnisse nicht vor 3 bis 5 Jahren nach Studienbeginn zu erwarten sind. Gerade die Prothetik braucht aber Langzeitbeobachtungen, um überhaupt sinnvolle Aussagen machen zu können (s. u.).*
– *Die Finanzkraft der Dentalindustrie ist nicht vergleichbar mit der pharmazeutischen Industrie; eine tatkräftige Förderung ist nur in engen Grenzen möglich.*
– *In der Zahnmedizin gilt das MPG – daher besteht keine Notwendigkeit von Phase II–IV-Studien.*
– *Der Generationswechsel der zahnmedizinischen Produkte wird bestimmt vom IDS-Rhythmus, die alle zwei Jahre stattfindet – meist ist ein Material schon vom Markt genommen, bevor klinische Forschungsergebnisse vorliegen.*
– *Zahnmedizin ist bei weitem nicht so spektakulär wie die Medizin.*

So zutreffend diese Aufzählung ist, so wenig ist sie geeignet, die Verantwortlichen aus ihrer Pflicht zu entlassen, sich wissenschaftlich mit den dringendsten Problemen ihres Fachgebietes auseinanderzusetzen.

6.4.2 Spezifische prothetische Probleme

Eine ganze Anzahl von fachspezifischen Problemen sorgt dafür, dass evidenz-basierte Leitlinien für die Prothetik nicht einfach zu entwickeln sein werden. Sie lassen sich in drei Punkten zusammenfassen:

– Bedarfsdefinition,
– multidimensionale Ergebnisbewertung,
– Zeitfaktor.

6.4.2.1 Prothetischer Bedarf

Normativer prothetischer Behandlungsbedarf (durch Zahnverlust) und subjektiver Bedarf (Zahnersatz) weichen weltweit erheblich voneinander ab, in dem Sinne, dass der Bedarf ungleich umfangreicher eingeschätzt wird als das Anliegen, sich Zahnersatz anfertigen zu lassen. Der normative Bedarf wäre wohl auch von keinem Gesundheitssystem der Welt zu decken. Hinzu kommt, dass über die „Anforderungsprothetik" zusätzliche Bereiche erschlossen werden, die sich der medizinischen Notwendigkeit entziehen (z. B. Behandlungen aus ästhetischen Motiven). Verantwortlich für dieses widersprüchliche Geschehen sind individuelle Faktoren, Lebensstil, soziale und kulturelle Umweltfaktoren (vgl. Walter et al., 1999; Bergman, 1999). Die Entscheidung für oder gegen Zahnersatz wird maßgeblich beeinflusst von der Steigerung an Lebensqualität, die sich der Patient davon erhofft. Als

Konsequenz daraus ergibt sich (vgl. Figgener, 1999): Es existieren viele unterschiedliche zahnmedizinisch-prothetische Antworten bei gleichem oder ähnlichem Befund und unterschiedlicher individueller Notwendigkeit. Evidenz-basierte Leitlinien auf der Basis des aktuellen wissenschaftlichen Erkenntnisstandes können dies vermutlich nur unzureichend reflektieren. Eine Eingrenzung über Zahnersatz-Richtlinien, wie sie derzeit existieren, erscheint jedoch im Zeitalter von EBD nicht adäquat.

6.4.2.2 Multidimensionale Ergebnisbewertung

Prothetische Behandlungsmaßnahmen müssen stets unter verschiedenen Sichtweisen bewertet werden (vgl. Guckes, Scurria und Shugars, 1996; Anderson, 1998): Neben seiner Langlebigkeit, über die schon berichtet wurde, weist Zahnersatz spezifische physiologische, psycho-soziale und ökonomische Effekte auf, die gegen Nichtbehandlung bzw. alternative Behandlungsstrategien abzuwägen sind. In der herkömmlichen Darstellung wird bisher zu wenig Rücksicht auf diese Tatsache genommen, vielmehr wird meist nur eine Wirkung hervorgehoben. Über die Wirksamkeit von Zahnersatz in seinen verschiedenen Ausführungsformen selbst wurden nur wenige Forschungsarbeiten unternommen.

6.4.2.3 Zeitfaktor

Für eine sachgerechte Beurteilung des prothetischen Ersatzes ist es unabdingbar, die während der Tragezeit des Ersatzes beobachtbaren Fakten zu sammeln und in eine korrekte Zuordnung zur Zeitspanne, die seit seiner Eingliederung vergangen ist, zu setzen. Laboruntersuchungen oder Computersimulationen können prothetisch-klinische Studien bisher in keiner Weise ersetzen. Langzeituntersuchungen bleiben also zunächst der „Königsweg", um in der zahnärztlichen Prothetik zu tragfähigen Erkenntnissen zu gelangen, die dem Patienten nützen. Dieses Vorgehen wird aber auch als besonders hinderlich für eine schnelle Material- und Methodenentwicklung angesehen (vgl. Krejci, 1992). Man mag dies bedauern, aber prothetische Maßnahmen haben weder eine vitale Indikation, noch sind die zu erwartenden Fortschritte so einschneidend, wie die Dentalindustrie dies glauben macht.

Zahlreiche Beispiele illustrieren, dass Jahre nach einer begeistert gefeierten Einführung eines neuen Werkstoffes Ernüchterung um sich greift. Ein typisches Beispiel bildet die Vollkeramik-Krone aus Dicor. Nach übereinstimmenden Berichten aus Deutschland und den USA waren bei Langzeituntersuchungen (vgl. Erpenstein und Kerschbaum, 1991; Borchard, Erpenstein und Kerschbaum, 1998; Malament und Socransky, 1999) nach mehr als 10 Jahren bereits mehr als ein Drittel aller Kronen zerstört – ein kaum vertretbarer Misserfolg im Vergleich zur klassischen Metallkeramik (ca. 10%

Misserfolg nach dieser Zeitperiode). Auch ausgereifte werkstoffkundliche Experimente schützen keineswegs vor klinischen Misserfolgen: Man denke an die Prognostizierbarkeit von Verfahren zur Prüfung des Metall-Kunststoffverbundes und die wenig übereinstimmenden klinischen Daten, die hierzu aus der Adhäsivprothetik existieren (vgl. Kerschbaum und Haastert, 1995).

Aus dem Gesagten lässt sich ableiten, dass Zahnersatz fast immer auf Langzeitwirkungen abzielt. Evidenz über den Wert einer prothetischen Versorgung kann daher auch erst nach einem längeren Zeitraum der Erprobung festgestellt werden (min. 5 Jahre).

6.5 Zusammenfassung

Die zahnärztliche Prothetik benötigt evidenz-basierte Leitlinien auf all ihren Gebieten. Bisher sind solche Leitlinien nicht verfügbar. Die zur Zeit akzeptierten Regeln (z. B. DGZMK-Statements) sind zwar wertvoll, aber nur auf Expertenniveau abgefasst. Dies liegt vor allem daran, dass das Evidenzniveau, auf dem die meisten klinisch bedeutsamen Entscheidungen in zahnärztlichen Fragestellungen beruhen, bescheiden ist: Randomisierte, kontrollierte Studien (RCTs) fehlen zu den meisten klinisch wichtigen Problemen fast völlig, Meta-Analysen sind bisher nur zu wenigen Fragestellungen veröffentlicht worden. Wichtigste aktuelle Erkenntnisquelle prothetischer Entscheidungen sind retrospektive Fall-Kontrollstudien, die reichlich vorliegen und auch lange Zeiträume (bis 15 Jahre) abdecken. Bis evidenzbasierte prothetische Leitlinien vorliegen werden, dürfte längere Zeit vergehen. Es ist Aufgabe der Fachgesellschaften (z. B. DGZPW), mit der Leitlinienentwicklung zu beginnen und unter strategischen Gesichtspunkten Themen auszuwählen.

Dank

Für die tatkräftige Unterstützung und Hilfe bei der Literatur- und Internetsuche möchte ich meinen Kollegen K. Böning (Dresden) und J. Türp (Freiburg) sehr herzlich danken.

6 Evidence-based dentistry as a basis of prosthetic therapy

Thomas Kerschbaum, Cologne

6.1 Preliminary note

Clinical decisions in prosthodontics are at present based predominantly on three factors: (1) the experience the individual dentist has been able to acquire in the exercise of his profession and/or can draw upon through his training and knowledge of publications; (2) the dentist's values and intuitions; and (3) the available resources (cf. Muir Gray, 1997). Within this triad, opinion-based decision-making on the appropriate prosthetic therapy has traditionally played the most important part. This approach may explain why similar clinical findings in relation to a patient's masticatory situation can lead to completely different therapy options that differ enormously in cost. However, owing to increasing pressure on available resources and the growing acceptance of comparative scientific studies of the various therapy options, it is now essential to promote evidence-based therapy decisions in prosthetics and thereby at the same time to apply quality assurance criteria.

Practising dentists and dental students in particular must surely be confused when they learn in their training about numerous "laws" and "rules", such as Ante's law, Thielemann's law, the Hanau Quint, Costen's syndrome and the Károlyi effect (cf. Türp & Antes, 2000), that seemingly lack any basis of scientific evidence. Critical views have been expressed on the minimal proportion of validly underpinned knowledge in the dental field: Böning (2000) quoted a figure of 8% and Marinello (1999) 10–15%, but the sources of these estimates are unspecified.

6.2 Why evidence-based decisions?

There are at present four main reasons to contemplate the development and introduction of evidence-based guidelines for dental prosthetics (cf. Böning, 2000, modified):

– Prosthetic measures are important for the quality of people's lives.
– Prosthodontic therapy results in high costs for the health system.

– Disproportionate differences in quality and cost exist between possible treatment options.
– There seems to be a need for improvement in the quality of treatment.

Dental prostheses are a significant determinant of our quality of life today, as current representative population statistics and surveys confirm (cf. Walter, Roediger & Rieger, 1999; Walter et al., 1999; IDZ, 1999; see Table 6-1). Taking all types of prosthetic therapy together, from single crowns to complete denture prostheses, more than 50% of the 35-44 age group already have some type of prosthesis – in other words, from this age group on, every other member of the population already has recourse to therapy of this kind. In the oldest age groups, almost every individual in the Federal Republic considers dental prostheses to be necessary (see Fig. 6-1) and regards them as particularly important to his or her quality of life. The reason is clear: despite all our prophylactic efforts and successes, typically 10–15 teeth are still lost in Germany today between the ages of 35 and 64. A quarter of the German population aged between 65 and 74 are currently edentulous and wear complete prostheses. Social norms and other considerations (aesthetics, speech and masticatory function) ensure that no one can escape the "compulsion" to wear dentures.

According to recent statistics, some 35% (nominal value approximately 11 billion DM) of total German dental expenditure in 1996 (about 35 billion DM) was accounted for by prosthodontics (projection of figures in Bauer, Neumann & Saekel, 1994). Dentistry currently makes up an appreciable

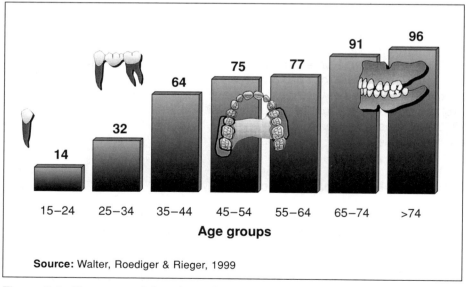

Figure 6-1: Frequency of dental prostheses (per cent)

6.2 Why evidence-based decisions?

Table 6-1: Prostheses in middle-aged and older subjects			
		Age 35–44	Age 65–74
		%	%
Partial prosthesis	UJ	5.8	28.3
Partial prosthesis	LJ	6.7	36.2
Complete prosthesis	UJ	2.1	41.8
Complete prosthesis	LJ	1.1	26.2
Complete prosthesis	UJ/LJ	1.1	24.0
Source: IDZ: DMS III, 1999			

proportion of total health costs in this country (some 550 billion DM per year). A typical household (in the west) must, according to the Federal Statistical Office (1998), budget on average for 536 DM of extra payments for dental prostheses – more than for any other sector of health expenditure (e. g. medicines).

Media reporting on the quality of dental care, and in particular of dental prostheses, tends to be sensational and usually negative (for example, the news magazine "Der Spiegel" reported on quality deficiencies in dental care, 12/1990; the study "Market transparency in prosthodontics" by the WIdO [Scientific Institute of the Local Health Insurance Funds], Bauer & Huber, 1999). For all the justified criticism levelled at such studies (cf. Walther & Meyer, 1999), it must be admitted that differences of opinion and uncertainties exist about the choice of the appropriate therapy based on the clinical findings. For example, every day dentists have to decide whether a given tooth is sound enough to be treated with a plastic (or cast) filling or whether a crown restoration is required: either there is no firm criterion for making this decision (cf. Covey et al., 1999; Staehle, 1999), or else the answers that exist are barely adequate. The question whether a crown or filling must be renewed or can be left as it is cannot at present be answered on the basis of clear, reliable criteria even though re-dentistry today probably accounts for the lion's share of the dental budget. The list of routine dental interventions on which opinions diverge could be extended almost ad infinitum. This also applies specifically to typical prosthetic problems: Figure 6-2 shows the six prosthetic treatment options for one missing anterior tooth (see Fig. 6-2); Figure 6-3 sets out the typical free-end treatment alternatives (see Fig. 6-3); and Table 6-2 compares costs and average survival rates (see Table 6-2).

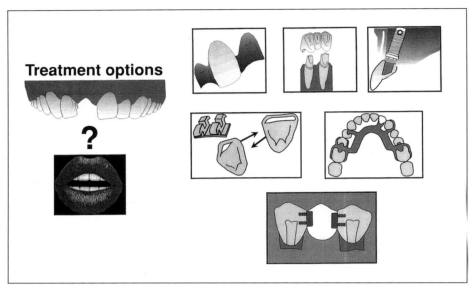

Figure 6-2: Treatment options for an anterior tooth edentulous space (adhesive bridge, conventional bridge, single implant, orthodontic space closure, partial prosthesis, UDA bridge [no longer indicated owing to increased susceptibility to caries at anchor point])

Table 6-2: Cost and average survival period of different forms of prosthetic appliances		
Appliance	Cost index	Survival (years)
Plastic prosthesis	0.2	3
Frame prosthesis	0.5	8
Adhesive bridge	0.5	10
Porcelain-fused-to-metal bridge	1.0	20
Single implant	1.6	20
Source: Öwall, Käyser & Carlsson, 1996, p. 14		

6.3 Sources of evidence in prosthetics

6.3.1 The Internet

Consultation of the typical Internet sources (NHS Centre for Reviews and Dissemination, University of York, The Cochrane Collaboration, Center for Evidence-Based Dentistry, Institute of Health, EBM/Ulm, AWMF[1] State-

---
[1] Association of Scientific and Medical Specialist Societies.

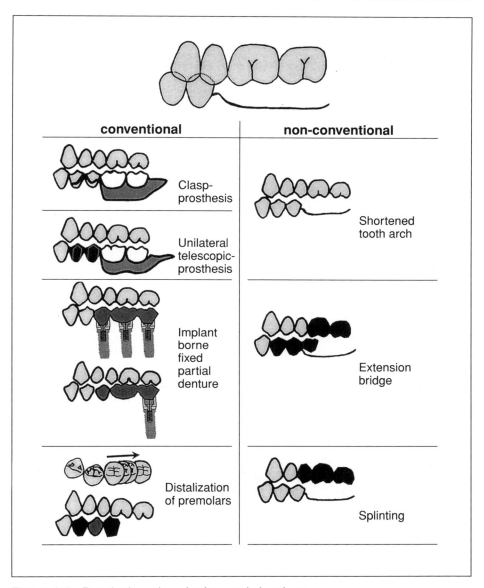

Figure 6-3: Prosthetic options for free-end situations

ments, Health Evidence Bulletins for Wales) using the search string "oral health" yields very little specific material on prosthodontics. Pathology of the temporomandibular joint and oro-facial pain syndrome are covered (also by the AWMF), and there is material on extreme tooth wear. However, no evidence-based prosthetic guidelines were found, even in rudimentary form.

6.3.2 Meta-analyses

A search for the term "meta-analysis" (search period: 1994 to 1999) in Medline resulted in 25 hits, of which only four related to prosthetic topics:

– veneers,
– bridge survival times (two hits),
– adhesive bridges.

6.3.2.1 Veneers

Evaluating a total of 39 studies on the use of ceramic and resin-based veneers dating from the period 1983 to 1996, Meijering (1997) and Kreulen, Creugers & Meijering (1998) concluded that the survival rate of ceramic veneers (n = 1552), at 92% after four years, was better than that of resin veneers (n = 323), of which only 78% were still surviving after three years.

6.3.2.2 Bridges

Long-term studies of dental clinics and practices based on systematic files and documentation (dental treatment records and insurance documentation) afford a virtually complete view of the durability – i.e. fate – of crowns and bridges after cementation. Nowadays, to be acceptable, all such material must be time-related (e.g. in the form of Kaplan-Meier statistics – cf. Kaplan & Meier, 1958). Tables 6-3 and 6-4 set out the results of two meta-analyses (cf. Creugers, Käyser & van't Hof, 1994; Scurria, Bader & Shugars, 1998) on the survival rate of fixed partial dentures and their abutments (see Tables 6-3 and 6-4). These results showed that two thirds of all bridges were still performing their therapeutic function after 15 years in place. Some 96–98% of all abutment teeth were still functional 10 years after therapy.

6.3.2.3 Adhesive bridges

Several studies with the character of meta-analyses exist on this subject. Creugers & van't Hof (1991) and Kerschbaum & Haastert (1995) found that adhesive bridges are indicated preferentially in young people with caries-free dentition for small edentulous spaces between sound teeth. They are very susceptible to complications in the post-treatment period: almost one bridge in two becomes detached at least once in 10 years.

6.3 Sources of evidence in prosthetics

Table 6-3: Survival of crowns and bridges – long-term results				
	Crowns			
First author	Year	Number	Time (years)	Survival rate (%)
Westermann	1990	222	8	88
Kerschbaum	1991	4371	15	59
Erpenstein	1992	593	15	84
BKK[2] study	1992	20946	6	94
Schlösser	1993	390	9	93
Langel	1994	112	8	89
Nordmeyer	1996	472	5	99
Stoll	1999	1679	10	86 (partial crowns)
	Bridges			
First author	Year	Number	Time (years)	Survival rate (%)
Leempoel	1987	1674	12	87
Kerschbaum	1991	1669	15	64
Erpenstein	1992	298	15	60
BKK study	1992	2578	6	97
Creugers	1994	Meta-analysis	15	74
Seth	1995	2583	10	76
Nordmeyer	1996	131	5	98
Scurria	1998	Meta-analysis	15	75
Source: Kerschbaum, 2000				

6.3.3 DGZMK[3] Statements

The DGZMK's Statements, which are published in Germany at irregular intervals, may certainly be deemed to possess the character of expert-level guidelines. Of the total of 88 current Statements (as at December 1999), however, only 11 covered prosthetic topics (see Table 6-5). Comparison of

---

[2] Federal Association of Corporate Health Insurance Funds.
[3] German Society of Dentistry and Oral Medicine.

Table 6-4: Survival of abutment teeth – long-term results

First author	Year	Crown/bridge abutments (number)	Time (years)	Survival rate (%)
Hain	1993	222	8	96 *(complete/ partial crowns)*
Schlösser	1993	390	9	99 *(complete crowns)*
Schlösser	1993	725	9	99 *(partial crowns)*
Schlösser	1993	588	9	96 *(bridges)*
Langel	1994	112	10	98 *(crowns)*
Seth	1995	3313	10	96 *(bridges)*
Scurria	1998	1525	10	96 *(bridges [porcelain fused to metal])*

Source: Kerschbaum, 2000

Table 6-5: Numbers of DGZMK Statements in dental specialties (as at December 1999)

Topics	n
General dentistry	31
Conservative dentistry	17
Prosthetics	11
Surgery	9
Periodontology	6
Preventive dentistry	8
Orthodontics	3
Radiology	3
Total	**88**

the DGZMK Statements with guideline-type publications by other specialized dental societies (e.g. the AWMF) shows that the DGZMK Statements in the prosthetic field are of undeniable competence and based on a solid foundation of evidence.

6.3.4 Specialist organizations in other countries (USA)

The very title "Parameters of Care" used by the American College of Prosthodontists (March 1996) for its 70-page paper indicates that this document was intended as a kind of guideline. It therefore covers all fields of activity in this specialty: the recording and evaluation of clinical findings, alterations in individual teeth, partial and total edentulousness, implant prosthetics, aesthetic prosthetics, treatment of patients with temporomandibular disorders, epithetics and maxillofacial prosthetics, treatment of sleep disturbances, local anaesthesia and adjuvant measures. The information given includes standards, diagnostic directives, therapeutic objectives, and risk factors. However, closer examination reveals nothing but a collation of chapter titles from textbooks. All the characterizing features of EBD are lacking. For example, the only criteria mentioned for deciding whether a crown restoration is necessary or filling is still feasible are loss of tooth hard tissue and its causes (caries, attrition, erosion, abfraction, fractures and infractions, or endodontic therapy).

6.4 Development of prosthetic guidelines: the problems

6.4.1 General

In many fields of dental activities, the difficulty of analysis is exacerbated by the enormous number of journals and papers currently published: every year some 42 000 dental articles appear worldwide in about 490 journals (cf. Spiekermann, 1999). It is therefore no longer possible to obtain an overview of specific topics or issues without search aids such as medical databases – e.g. Medline.

However, quality proves to be a more important problem than quantity: in a review of the three important international prosthetic journals (Journal of Prosthetic Dentistry, International Journal of Prosthodontic Dentistry and Journal of Prosthodontic Dentistry), Dumbrigue, Jones & Esquivel (1999 a & b) found that only 62 out of a total of 3631 articles were randomized clinically controlled studies (RCTs). This means that at most 1.7% of all international articles on prosthetic subjects achieved the highest level of evidence. As long ago as in 1996, Windeler was already disappointed to find that the studies in the leading German journals such as the Deutsche Zahnärztliche Zeitschrift (41%), as well as the Journal of Dental Research (20%) and Journal of Clinical Periodontology (75%) in the USA, were patient-oriented. A far smaller proportion of these studies conformed to the rules of "good clinical practice" (GCP).

A comparison of specialties by Badovinac, Conway & Niederman (1999) showed that significantly fewer RCTs (randomized controlled clinical studies) and MAs (meta-analyses) were published in the dental field than in specific medical specialties or disciplines (cardiology, gastroenterology, infectiology, dermatology, musculoskeletal diseases, endocrinology and haematology).

Böning (2000) speculated on the reasons for this deplorably low level in dentistry and, in particular, prosthetics:

- *The heavy burden of teaching ties up considerable resources; in addition, patients have to be treated and there are organizational problems.*
- *The "publish or perish" principle is increasingly shaping the landscape of dental research; long-term studies are no longer conducted because results cannot be expected until three to five years after commencement. However, prosthetics in particular needs long-term observations if meaningful results are to be forthcoming (see below).*
- *The financial muscle of the dental industry cannot be compared with that of the pharmaceutical sector; the potential for effective funding is therefore limited.*
- *The Medicinal Products Law (MPG) applies to dentistry in Germany, so that there is no need for Phase II-IV studies.*
- *The life of a generation of dental products is determined by the two-year cycle of the International Dental Show (IDS): materials are usually withdrawn from the market before clinical research results are available.*
- *Dentistry is far less spectacular than medicine.*

Spectacular as this enumeration is, it does not exonerate those responsible from their duty of engaging scientifically with the most urgent problems of their fields of specialization.

6.4.2 Specific prosthetic problems

Owing to a number of problems specific to the field, the development of evidence-based guidelines for prosthetics will not be a simple matter. These problems can be summarized under three headings:

- definition of treatment needs,
- multidimensional assessment of results,
- time factor.

6.4.2.1 Prosthetic treatment needs

Throughout the world the normative prosthetic treatment needs (based on tooth loss) differs substantially from the subjective demand (dental prostheses) in that the former is estimated to be incomparably greater than the wish of individual patients to have a prosthesis made. It is unlikely that the normative requirement could be covered by any health system in the world.

Moreover, the subjective demand for prostheses extends also to fields unconnected with medical necessity (e.g. aesthetically motivated treatment). These contradictions are attributable to individual variables, lifestyles, and social and cultural environmental factors (cf. Walter et al., 1999; Bergman, 1999). The decision pro or contra prosthetic therapy is substantially determined by the patient's hoped-for quality-of-life enhancement. Consequently (cf. Figgener, 1999), there are many possible prosthodontic responses to identical or similar clinical findings, according to differences in individual needs. Evidence-based guidelines in accordance with the current scientifically established state of the art probably cannot reflect this situation adequately. However, any restriction by prosthodontic directives of the type currently existing seems inappropriate in the age of EBD.

6.4.2.2 Multidimensional assessment of results

Prosthetic treatment measures must always be assessed by a combination of criteria (cf. Guckes, Scurria & Shugars, 1996; Anderson, 1998): in addition to its life, as already discussed, a prosthesis has specific physiological, psychosocial and economic effects, which must be weighed against leaving the patient untreated or alternative treatment strategies. Too little attention has traditionally been paid to this aspect, the emphasis instead usually being placed on a single factor. There have been very few research projects on the efficacy of prosthetic dental treatment in all its various forms.

6.4.2.3 Time factor

A dental prosthesis can be validly assessed only if the observable facts are gathered throughout the period when it is worn and correctly correlated with the period that has elapsed since fitting. Laboratory investigations or computer simulations have so far proved no substitute for clinical prosthetic studies. In the prosthodontic field, therefore, long-term studies for the time being remain the royal road to obtaining valid results useful to the patient. This approach is, however, also regarded as a particular obstacle to the rapid development of materials and methods (cf. Krejci, 1992). Regrettable as it may seem, prosthetic measures do not have vital indications, nor are the advances to be expected as far-reaching as the dental industry would have us believe.

There are many examples where the introduction of a new material has met with an enthusiastic response, only to be followed some years later by the spread of a more sober view. The Dicor all-ceramic crown is typical. Reports of long-term studies from Germany and the USA (cf. Erpenstein & Kerschbaum, 1991; Borchard, Erpenstein & Kerschbaum, 1998; Malament & Socransky, 1999) agree that more than a third of all crowns had failed after more than 10 years, an unacceptable failure rate compared with classical porcelain fused to metal (about 10% failure after the same period). Even sophisticated experimentation using the techniques of materials science affords no protection from clinical failure: one need only consider the predictability of testing techniques for resin-bonded bridges and the divergent clinical data on these from the field of adhesive prosthetics (cf. Kerschbaum & Haastert 1995).

It is clear from the foregoing that dental prostheses are almost always intended to have long-term effects. Evidence on the value of a prosthetic measure can therefore accrue only after an extended trial period (not less than five years).

6.5 Summary

Evidence-based guidelines are needed in all fields of dental prosthetics. Such guidelines are not yet available. Although the currently accepted rules (e. g. DGZMK Statements) are valuable, they have been drawn up at expert level only. This is mainly because the level of evidence on which most clinically significant decisions in the dental field are taken is modest: randomized controlled studies (RCTs) are almost completely lacking on most clinically important problems, while meta-analyses have hitherto been published on only a few issues. The principal sources of information for prosthetic decisions at present are retrospective case control studies, which exist in large numbers and also cover long periods (up to 15 years). It will probably be a long time before evidence-based prosthetic guidelines are published. It is up to the specialized organizations (e. g. the DGZPW [German Society for Prosthodontics and Dental Material Science]) to commence the development of guidelines and to select topics according to strategic criteria.

Acknowledgements

I wish to express my warmest thanks to my colleagues K. Böning (Dresden) and J. Türp (Freiburg) for their active support and assistance with literature and Internet searching.

6.6 Literatur/References

American College of Prosthodontics: Parameters of Care. POC Version 1, March 1996. J Prosthodont 5 (1996), 1–70

Anderson, D. J.: The need for criteria on reporting treatment outcomes. J Prosthet Dent 79 (1998), 49–55

Badovinac, R., Conway, S., Niederman, R.: Bibliometric analysis of evidence-based dental therapeutics literature. J Dent Res 78, 124 (1999) Abstr. 148

Bauer, J., Neumann, T., Saekel, R.: Mundgesundheit und zahnmedizinische Versorgung in der Bundesrepublik Deutschland 1994. Berlin 1994

Bauer, J., Huber, H.: Markttransparenz beim Zahnersatz. Institut für angewandte Verbraucherforschung e.V./Wissenschaftliches Institut der AOK, Bonn (1999)

Bergman, B.: Die Zukunft der Prothetischen Zahnheilkunde. Editorial Dtsch Zahnärztl Z 54 (1999), 293–297

BKK Bundesverband der Betriebskrankenkassen: Qualität und Wirtschaftlichkeit in der zahnmedizinischen Versorgung. Essen 1992

Böning, K.: Leitlinien in der Zahnmedizin? In: Walter, M., Böning, K. Kongressband zum Mundgesundheitsworkshop Freiburg 1999, ISBN 3-89783-2 (erscheint 2/2000; will be published 2/2000)

Borchard, R., Erpenstein, H., Kerschbaum, T.: Langzeitverweildauer von galvanokeramischen und glaskeramischen (Dicor) Einzelkronen unter klinischen Bedingungen. DGZPW Vortrag in Leipzig (1998)

Covey, D. A., Kent, D. K., Dunning, D. G., Koka, S.: Qualitative and quantitative determination of dental amalgam restoration volume. J Prosthet Dent 82 (1999), 8–14

Creugers, N. H. J., van't Hof, M. A.: An analysis of clinical studies on resin bonded bridges. J Dent Res 70 (1991), 146–149

Creugers, N. H. J., Käyser, A. F., van't Hof, M. A.: A meta-analysis of durability data on conventional fixed bridges. Community Dent Oral Epidemiol 22 (1994), 448

Dumbrigue, H. B., Jones, J. S., Esquivel, J. F.: Evaluating Medline search strategies for randomized controlled trials in prosthodontics. J Dent Res 78, 144 (1999a) Ref. 307

Dumbrigue, H. B., Jones, J. S., Esquivel, J. F.: Developing a register of randomized controlled trials in prosthodontics. J Dent Res 78 (1999b), 144, Abstr. 308

Erpenstein, H., Kerschbaum, T.: Frakturrate von Dicor-Kronen unter klinischen Bedingungen. Dtsch Zahnärztl Z 46 (1991), 6

Erpenstein, H., Kerschbaum, T., Fischbach, H.: Verweildauer und klinische Befunde bei Kronen und Brücken. Dtsch Zahnärztl Z 47 (1992), 315

Figgener, L.: Leitlinien zur Qualitätssicherung in der zahnprothetischen Versorgung. In: Leitlinien zur Qualitätssicherung in der zahnprothetischen Versorgung. Symposium des AOK-Bundesverbandes am 21.10.1999, 89 ff

Guckes, A. D., Scurria, M. S., Shugars, D. A.: A conceptual framework for understanding of oral implant therapy. J Prosthet Dent 75 (1996), 633–639

Hain, H.: Die Verweildauer von extensiven Amalgamrestaurationen in einer zahnärztlichen Praxis. Med Diss Köln (1993)

IDZ, Institut der Deutschen Zahnärzte (Hrsg.): Dritte Deutsche Mundgesundheitsstudie (DMS III). Köln 1999

Kaplan, E. L., Meier, P.: Nonparametric estimation from incomplete observations. J Am Stat Ass 53 (1958), 457

Kerschbaum, T., Paszyna, C., Klapp, S., Meyer, G.: Verweilzeit und Risikofaktorenanalyse von festsitzendem Zahnersatz. Dtsch Zahnärztl Z 46 (1991), 20

Kerschbaum, T., Haastert, B.: Nachuntersuchungsergebnisse. In: Kerschbaum, T. (Hrsg.): Adhäsivprothetik. München 1995

Kerschbaum, T.: Ergebnisorientierte Versorgung mit Kronen und Brücken. In: Heidemann, D. (Hrsg.): Deutscher Zahnärztekalender 2000. Köln, München 2000

Krejci, I.: Zahnfarbene Restaurationen. München 1992

Kreulen, C. M., Creugers, N. H. J., Meijering, A. C.: Meta-analysis of anterior veneer restorations in clinical studies. J Dent 26 (1998), 345–353

Langel, W. Ch.: Extensive Amalgamfüllungen im Vergleich zu Einzelkronen – eine Longitucinalstudie. Med Diss, Köln 1994

Leempoel, P. J. B.: Levensduur en Nabehandelingen van Kronen en conventionele Bruggen in de algemeine praktijk. Thesis, Nijmegen (NL) 1987

Leempoel, P. J. B., Käyser, A. F., van Rossum, G. M. J. M., de Haan, A. F. J.: The survival rate of bridges. A study of 1674 bridges in 40 Dutch general practices. J Oral Rehabil 22 (1995), 327

Malament, K. A., Socransky, S. S.: Survival of Dicor glass-ceramic dental restorations over 14 years: Part I: Survival of Dicor complete coverage restorations and effect of internal surface acid etching, tooth position, gender, and age. J Prosthet Dent 81 (1999), 23–32

Marinello, C. P.: Klinik für Prothetik und Kaufunktionslehre. In: *Vauthier, Th.:* Basel ein Standbein der Zahnmedizin in der Schweiz. Schweiz Mschr Zahnmed 109 (1999), 1216–1221

Meijering, C.: A clinical study on veneer restorations. Habilitationsschrift. Nijmegen 1997

Muir Gray, J. A.: Evidence-based healthcare. New York 1997

Nordmeyer, J.: Verweildaueranalyse und klinische Nachuntersuchung von festsitzendem Zahnersatz unter besonderer Berücksichtigung der Kronenrandspaltbreiten. Med Diss, Köln 1996

Öwall, B., Käyser, A. F., Carlsson, G. E.: Prosthodontics – principles and management strategies. Mosby-Wolfe, London 1996

Schlösser, R.: Longitudinale Untersuchung von festsitzendem Zahnersatz – Teilkrone und Vollgusskronen im Vergleich. Med Diss, Köln 1993

Schlösser, R., Kerschbaum, T., Ahrens, F. J., Cramer, M.: Überlebensrate von Teil- und Vollgusskronen. Dtsch Zahnärztl Z 48 (1993), 696

6.6 Literatur/References

Scurria, M. S., Bader, J. D., Shugars, D. A.: Meta-analysis of fixed partial denture survival: Prosthesis and abutments. J Prosthet Dent 79 (1998), 459–464

Seth, M.: Verweildaueranalyse von Brücken und Kronenblocks einer Kassenpraxis unter besonderer Berücksichtigung der Verblendung. Med Diss, Köln 1995

Der Spiegel, Nachrichtenmagazin, Hamburg Heft 12/1990

Spiekermann, J.: Number of Dental Publications. Pers. Mitt/personal communication (1999)

Staehle, H. J.: Abgrenzung zwischen konservierender und prothetischer Behandlungsnotwendigkeit. In: Leitlinien zur Qualitätssicherung in der zahnprothetischen Versorgung. Symposium des AOK Bundesverbandes am 21. 10. 1999. 69 ff

Stoll, R., Siewecke, M., Pieper, K., Stachniss, V., Schulte, A.: Longevity of cast gold inlays and partial crowns – a retrospective study at a dental school clinic. Clin Oral Invest 3 (1999), 100–104

Türp, J. C., Antes, G.: Evidenzbasierte Zahnmedizin. Dtsch Zahnärztl Z (im Druck/in print)

Walter, M., Roediger, J., Rieger, Ch.: Bevölkerungsrepräsentative zahnärztliche-prothetische Studie: Versorgungsgrad im Bundesland Sachsen. Dtsch Zahnärztl Z 54 (1999), 25–30

Walter, M., Böning, K., Schütte, U., v. Majewski, J., Kordaß, B., Müller, N., Scheller, H., Stark, H.: Bestimmung des zahnärztlich-prothetischen Behandlungsbedarfs. Teil 1/Teil 2. Zahnärztl Welt, 108 (1999), 449–453 und 522–526

Walther, W., Meyer, V. P.: Dem wissenschaftlichen Anspruch nicht gerecht. Zahnärztl Mitt 17 (1999), 20–23

Westermann, W., Kerschbaum, Th., Hain, H.: Verweildauer von ausgedehnten Amalgamfüllungen. Dtsch Zahnärztl Z 45 (1990), 743–747

Windeler, J.: Mehr klinische Forschung in der Zahnmedizin. Editorial Dtsch Zahnärztl Z 51 (1996), 69

7 Evidenz-basierte Zahnheilkunde in der Kariestherapie

Elmar Reich, Homburg/Saar

7.1 Vorbemerkung

Die Grundlagen der evidenz-basierten Medizin wurden erst in den letzten Jahren beschrieben. Das Ziel dabei ist nicht eine andere Wissenschaftlichkeit, sondern nach Sackett et al. (1996): „der gewissenhafte, ausdrückliche und vernünftige Gebrauch der gegenwärtig besten externen, wissenschaftlichen Evidenz für Entscheidungen über die medizinische Versorgung individueller Patienten."

Daraus könnte man für die evidenz-basierte Zahnerhaltung ableiten, „die sinnvolle Anwendung einer umfassenden Diagnose und Intervention zur Erhaltung der Zähne und des Zahnhalteapparates des Patienten" (vgl. McGuire und Nunn, 1996).

Vor kurzem hat in Deutschland eine Studie (vgl. Bauer und Huber, 1999) bei Erwachsenen in Zahnarztpraxen für Aufsehen gesorgt, weil sich die Therapiepläne und die Kosten bei verschiedenen Zahnärzten für denselben Patienten sehr stark unterschieden haben. Analog wurden im Readers Digest (vgl. Eckenberg, 1997) Therapiepläne vorgestellt, die von 50 Zahnärzten in den USA aufgestellt worden waren und die zwischen 500 und 30000 $ schwankten.

Die Erwartungen, die an eine evidenz-basierte Zahnerhaltung gestellt werden, beziehen sich auf

– die individuelle Versorgung mit einer Verbesserung der Qualität, der Lebensdauer sowie der Funktion und Ästhetik der zahnärztlichen Versorgung,
– Verbesserungen im zahnärztlichen Gesundheitssystem, die über eine Verbesserung der Qualität sowie eine Reduktion der Kosten charakterisiert werden.

Es soll nun in den folgenden drei Bereichen der Zahnerhaltung die vorhandene Evidenz überprüft werden:

- Kariesdiagnose,
- Prävention,
- Therapie.

7.2 Evidenz in der Kariesdiagnose

Bei der größten zahnärztlich-wissenschaftlichen Tagung, durchgeführt von der International Association for Dental Research/IADR (vgl. J Dent Res, 1999), wurde die weitaus überwiegende Zahl von wissenschaftlichen Arbeiten aus dem Bereich der Materialkunde und Füllungstherapie präsentiert, weit abgeschlagen gefolgt von Präventionsmaßnahmen und von Untersuchungen zur Kariesdiagnose. Eine medizinische Kariesdiagnose besteht aber nicht nur in der Detektion der Karies mittels Sonde oder anderer Hilfsmittel (vgl. Reich, 1997; Lussi, 1998; von Ohle und Reich, 1997). Daneben sollte eine Bestimmung des Kariesrisikos durchgeführt werden (vgl. Reich, Lussi und Newbrun, 1999). Aufbauend auf diese Befunde kann der individuelle Interventionsbedarf für jeden Patienten (vgl. Benn und Melzer, 1998; Edelstein, 1994; Berkey, Shay und Holm-Pedersen, 1996) bestimmt werden.

Die Sensitivität und Spezifität verschiedener Verfahren zur Kariesdiagnose wurde mittels aufwendiger Studien (vgl. Lussi et al., 1999; Verdonschot et al., 1999) bestimmt. Abhängig von der Lokalisation der Karies zeigt es sich, dass visuelle Verfahren und die Anwendung der Sonde nur eine Sensitivität von ca. 50% besitzen. Röntgenologische Verfahren bringen nur eine geringfügige Verbesserung der durchschnittlichen Leistung. Weitere technische Verfahren, wie z. B. die faseroptische Transillumination (FOTI), sind auch nicht in der Lage, die Diagnose wesentlich zu verbessern. Besser geeignet sind hingegen das Laser-Fluoreszenzverfahren (vgl. Lussi et al., 1999; Abb. 7-1) oder die elektrische Impedanzmessung (ERM; vgl. Verdonschot et al., 1999).

Für den Approximalbereich stellen nach Korrektur der Befunde auf klinische Fehldiagnosen hin Röntgenverfahren die bisher sicherste Methode dar (vgl. Verdonschot et al., 1999; Abb. 7-2). Keine wesentlichen Verbesserungen erbrachten visuelle Untersuchungen oder Untersuchungen mit der Sonde oder FOTI. Erste Ergebnisse mit der Laserfluoreszenz zeigten aber auch für Approximalflächen ein vielversprechendes Potenzial (vgl. Longbottom et al., 1999a; Eggertsson et al., 1999; Wagner, Longbottom und Pitts, 1999).

Als Goldstandard für die Kariesdiagnose werden meist Demineralisationen oder Kavitationen im Dentinbereich (vgl. Ekstrand et al., 1998; Longbottom et al., 1999b) angegeben. Dieser Goldstandard muss aber kritisch evaluiert werden, da er nicht die Feststellung des Interventionsbedarfs für Initialläsionen zulässt, insbesondere dort, wo Prophylaxemaßnahmen noch in der Lage sind, das Fortschreiten der Karies zu stoppen (vgl. Pitts und Longbottom, 1995; Pine und ten Bosch, 1996; Reich, 1997; von Ohle und Reich,

7.2 Evidenz in der Kariesdiagnose

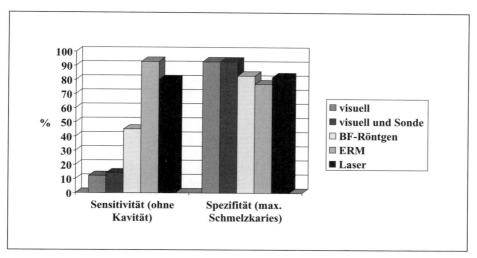

Abbildung 7-1: Sensivität und Spezifität verschiedener Methoden zur Diagnose der Okklusalkaries (vgl. Lussi et al., 1999)

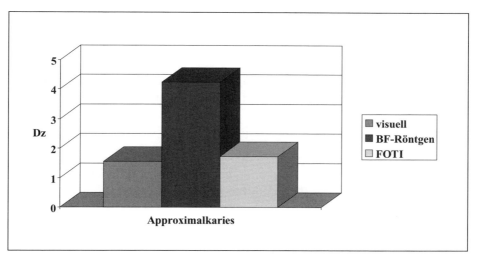

Abbildung 7-2: Durchschnittliche Fähigkeit (Dz) verschiedener diagnostischer Methoden für die Diagnose der Approximalkaries (vgl. Verdonschot et al., 1999)

1997). Schon bei einer sorgfältigen klinischen Diagnose sind initiale Demineralisationen im Schmelzbereich erkennbar, sie sind in Deutschland bei 12-Jährigen 8-mal häufiger als kariesbedingte Kavitäten im Dentin (vgl. Schiffner und Reich, 1999). Insofern muss die Standarddiagnose nach der Definition „Karies gleich Kavität" geändert werden. Gerade in der zahnärztlichen Praxis muss eine umfassende medizinische Diagnose der Karies durchgeführt werden. Der Bedarf an Intervention teilt sich dann auf in Restauration, kombiniert mit Prävention für kariöse Kavitäten, sowie Maßnahmen der Individualprophylaxe, wenn klinisch nur Initialläsionen oder mittels technischer Systeme Demineralisationen nachweisbar sind (vgl. Pitts und Kidd, 1992; Pitts und Longbottom, 1995; Lussi, 1999; Netuschil, Dahmen und Reich, 1999).

Die Risikobestimmungen für die Parodontitis (vgl. Page und Beck, 1997) und die Karies (vgl. Reich, Lussi und Newbrun, 1999) sind neue Verfahren, die noch relativ große Unsicherheiten aufweisen. Die Anwendung kommerzieller mikrobiologischer Tests oder Speicheltests alleine, ohne die Bewertung klinischer Faktoren, ist aber nicht ausreichend, um das Erkrankungsrisiko für die Therapieplanung präzise genug bestimmen zu können.

Nach einer umfassenden medizinischen Kariesdiagnose kann somit in der Praxis der Interventionsbedarf für präventive oder invasive Maßnahmen bestimmt werden. Da zuviel Interventionen eine Überbehandlung und damit unnötige Kosten bedeuten würden, muss der Bedarf aufgrund einer medizinischen Diagnose bestimmt werden. Negative Auswirkungen von Präventionsmaßnahmen sowohl durch den Patienten selbst als auch professionell in der Praxis, sind allerdings kaum zu erwarten. Anders sieht die Situation hingegen bei invasiven Therapien aus (vgl. Elderton und Mjör, 1992), wo unnötige Füllungen zu Folgeschäden für den Zahn oder – aufgrund von Nebenwirkungen – für den gesamten Organismus führen können. Recht uneinheitlich wird die Therapieplanung nach Kariesdiagnose durchgeführt (vgl. Amer et al., 1998; Tveit, Espelid und Skodje, 1999).

Ein schwerwiegendes und wissenschaftlich noch unbefriedigend gelöstes Problem ist die Diagnose der Sekundärkaries und die Feststellung des Erneuerungsbedarfs von Restaurationen (vgl. Kidd, 1996; Mjör, 1981; Jokstad et al., im Druck). In Industrienationen mit funktionierendem zahnärztlichen Versorgungssystem stellt die Erneuerung von Restaurationen mit ca. 60% (vgl. Chadwick et al., 1999) einen sehr großen Teil aller Restaurationsmaßnahmen dar. Die Lebensdauer einer Restauration wird jedoch meist durch den Zahnarzt bestimmt, da dieser die Diagnose bezüglich der Erneuerung (vgl. Tveit und Espelid, 1992) einer Restauration stellt. Alternativen stellen heute auch kostengünstigere und weniger invasive Verfahren, wie die Reparatur von Füllungen (vgl. Ettinger, 1990; Mjör, 1993) oder zusätzliche Versiegelungen, dar.

7.3 Evidenz in der Prävention

In der letzten Zeit (vgl. Ashley et al., 1999; CDA, 1999; ten Cate, 1999) wurde der Effekt der Fluoride präziser bestimmt und festgestellt, dass

7.3 Evidenz in der Prävention

- für Fluoridkonzentration und Kariesreduktion eine Dosis/Wirkungsbeziehung besteht,
- zwischen der Häufigkeit des Zähneputzens und der Kariesreduktion eine positive Korrelation vorhanden ist,
- Nachspülen mit Wasser nach dem Zähneputzen die Kariesreduktion negativ beeinflusst,
- zwischen der Menge an Zahnpaste und der Kariesreduktion keine eindeutige Korrelation besteht.

Die kariespräventive Wirkung von Fluoriden wurde in vielen Untersuchungen nachgewiesen. Dennoch sind unterschiedliche Empfehlungen über die Anwendung der Fluoride gemacht worden (vgl. WHO, 1994; CDA, 1994; CDA, 1999), und es stehen mehrere Überprüfungen der Evidenz der bestmöglichen Anwendung der Fluoride kurz vor dem Abschluss.

Die Konsensus-Konferenz der kanadischen Zahnärztegesellschaft (vgl. CDA, 1999) ist bezüglich der täglichen Fluoridanwendung zu folgenden Schlussfolgerungen (vgl. Tab. 7-1) mit entsprechenden Evidenzniveaus (vgl. Canadian Task Force, 1988) gekommen:

Tabelle 7-1: Konsensus-Konferenz der CDA – Schlussfolgerungen zur täglichen Fluoridanwendung	
1. Die Fluoridwirkung ist überwiegend topisch.	Evidenzniveau II-3
2. Die Wasserfluoridierung ist aufgrund ihres topischen Effektes effektiv.	Evidenzniveau II
3. Fluoridierte Zahnpasta stellt ein effektives Mittel dar, Fluoride topisch zu applizieren.	Evidenzniveau I
4. Das Verschlucken von mehr als der empfohlenen täglichen Fluoriddosis erhöht das Risiko für eine Dentalfluorose.	Evidenzniveau II-2
5. Werden keine topischen Fluoride in ausreichender Menge angewandt, insbesondere keine Fluoridzahnpasta oder fluoridiertes Trinkwasser, so sollten zusätzliche Fluoridprodukte in Form von Spüllösungen, Kautabletten oder Tropfen angewendet werden. Die Wirksamkeit dieser Fluoridprodukte ist – bei Schulkindern gering – und bei Kleinkindern nur selten untersucht.	 Evidenzniveau II-2 Evidenzniveau II-3
6. Bei einem sehr hohen Kariesrisiko kann die Verwendung topischer Fluoride allein nicht ausreichend sein, um Karies zu verhüten. Zusätzliche Fluoridanwendung kann nur einen geringen Effekt haben und andere Maßnahmen, wie z. B. die antimikrobielle Therapie und Veränderungen der Ernährung, können notwendig sein.	Evidenzniveau III
Quelle: CDA, 1999	

Im Rahmen der Ernährung können auch zuckerfreie Kaugummis die Kariesprophylaxe unterstützen (vgl. Imfeld, 1999).

Eine Fissurenversiegelung ist eine wirksame Maßnahme, um eine okklusale Karies zu verhüten. Die Zahlen für die Wirksamkeit der Fissurenversiegelung schwanken allerdings, da sie von der Kariesprävalenz, dem Kariesrisiko und auch der Retention des Versiegelungsmaterials abhängen. Nach 7 Jahren wurde in der Studie von Mertz-Fairhurst und Mitarbeitern (1984) über 50% Kariesreduktion ermittelt, wobei die Retentionsrate bei 66% lag. Nach 15 Jahren (vgl. Simonsen, 1991) wurden in 31% der ursprünglich versiegelten Flächen Karies oder Restaurationen gefunden, während dies bei den nicht versiegelten Flächen in 83% der Fall war. Verschiedene klinische Studien haben gezeigt, dass gerade auch bei kariesanfälligen Kindern die Versiegelung deutliche kariespräventive Effekte besitzt (vgl. Straffon und Dennison, 1988). Notwendig ist jedoch die Kontrolle und evtl. Nachversiegelung von Flächen, bei denen das Versiegelungsmaterial verloren gegangen ist. Jedoch fehlen nach Mitchell und Murray (1989) immer noch Studien, die die Kosteneffektivität der Versiegelung umfassend beweisen. Gerade in Deutschland sind die erst seit wenigen Jahren bei Kindern im GKV-Rahmen durchführbaren Versiegelungen wesentlich für den beobachteten Kariesrückgang (vgl. Abb. 7-3; Reich, 1999; Schiffner und Reich, 1999). Die Retentionsrate von Versiegelungen wie von Amalgamfüllungen an den Molaren bei 5- bis 8-jährigen Kindern beträgt nach Mitchell und Murray (1989) nur ungefähr zwei Jahre, was allerdings wohl als ein spezielles Problem der Kinderbehandlung aufgefasst werden muss.

Andere Methoden, wie die Applikation von Fluoriden (vgl. Stephen, 1995) oder antibakteriellen Produkten (vgl. Petersson, Netuschil und Brecx, im

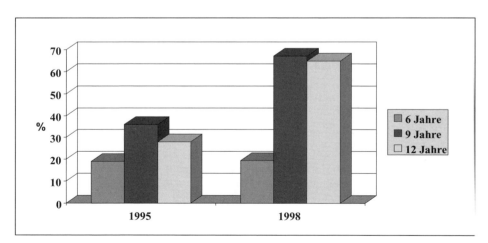

Abbildung 7-3: Anteil Versiegelungen an Molaren bayerischer Kinder (vgl. Reich, 1999)

Druck), können im Einzelfall durchaus positiv sein und ausreichen, um die Karies zu verhüten. Dies muss jedoch kontrolliert werden (Karies-Monitoring). Auch die Applikation von Glasionomerzementen ist nach Seppä und Forss (1991) und nach eigenen Studien viel versprechend. Für die dauerhafte Prävention sind kostengünstige, aber effektive Techniken in Kombination mit einer nach individuellen Risikokriterien bestimmten Versiegelung sinnvoll (vgl. Carvalho, Thylsturp und Ekstrand, 1992; Bader und Shugars, 1993). Die Bedeutung der Mundgesundheitserziehung für die Zahngesundheit wird generell als fraglich eingeschätzt (vgl. Kay und Locker, 1996). Von nachgewiesener Bedeutung sind die Hinweise zur Fluoridanwendung. Individuelle Gesundheitserziehung am Patientenstuhl scheint effektiver zu sein als über Massenmedien.

7.4 Evidenz in der Therapie

Das Postulat der „vollständigen" Entfernung kariösen Dentins wird seit den Anfängen der wissenschaftlichen Zahnheilkunde befolgt. Dennoch sollte man auch in der Therapie lange angewandte Konzepte oder Dogmen hinterfragen. Folgende Bereiche können analysiert werden:

– Kariestherapie,
– Indikation plastischer Füllungsmaterialien,
– Entscheidung Füllung oder Inlay/Krone.

Das Dogma der Kariesentfernung wird bewusst oder unbewusst in der Praxis nicht immer befolgt. So ist aufgrund der Schwierigkeiten der Kariesdiagnose („hidden caries") davon auszugehen, dass bis zu 35% kariöse Fissuren (vgl. Weerheijm et al., 1990; Weerheijm, Groen und Poorterman, 1999; Ricketts et al., 1997) trotz Dentinkaries versiegelt werden. In der Zwischenzeit liegt eine Studie über 10 Jahre vor (vgl. Mertz-Fairhurst et al., 1998), bei der unter klinisch kontrollierten Bedingungen eine Dentinkaries entweder entfernt und mit einer konventionellen Amalgamfüllung versehen wurde oder die Dentinkaries belassen wurde und die Kavität mit chemisch-härtendem Komposit und einer zusätzlichen Fissurenversiegelung versehen wurde. Als Ergänzung wurde eine Gruppe von Amalgamfüllungen ebenfalls zusätzlich versiegelt. Die Ergebnisse nach 10 Jahren zeigen, dass es auch bei der belassenen Karies und einer bakteriendichten Versorgung nur selten zu einer irreversiblen Pulpitis gekommen war. Die Misserfolgsquote für versiegelte Kompositfüllungen und klassische Amalgamfüllungen lag vergleichbar hoch.

Die Indikationsstellung für plastische Füllungsmaterialien ist aufgrund der Vielzahl angebotener Materialien und der Forderung des Patienten nach ästhetischen Füllungsmaterialien nicht einfach. Die jüngsten Analysen haben gezeigt, dass nach der bisher vorliegenden Evidenz Amalgamfüllungen als langlebigstes und billigstes Füllungsmaterial angesehen werden müssen (vgl. Chadwick et al., 1999). Hinzu kommt, dass oft neue restaurative Materialien auf den Markt gebracht werden, ohne dass eine ausreichende klinische Nachkontrolle durch wissenschaftliche Studien (vgl. Roulet, 1997) vorliegt. Die Auswertung von 195 Studien (vgl. Chadwick et al., 1999), die Kriterien für den Ersatz der Füllungen angegeben haben und entweder als prospektiv longitudinale Kohortenstudien oder als randomisierte klinische Studien durchgeführt wurden, zeigte, dass

– Amalgam langlebiger erscheint als Komposit,
– nur geringe Unterschiede zwischen Komposit/Keramik-Inlays vorhanden waren,
– die Kosteneffektivität von Amalgamfüllungen besser war als die adhäsiver Kompositfüllungen oder adhäsiver Inlays.

Einschränkend muss hier allerdings angemerkt werden, dass die zur Verfügung stehenden klinischen Studien mit Kompositen sich methodisch und bezüglich der Beobachtungszeit von solchen mit Amalgam unterschieden.

Ein weiterer Kritikpunkt bei vielen Studien betraf die meist fehlenden objektiven Parameter zur Feststellung der Qualität und der Lebensdauer. Die Kriterien für die Erneuerung von Füllungen waren meist nicht exakt definiert und dadurch wurde zweifellos die Funktionsdauer reduziert, wodurch wiederum nicht die mögliche Lebensdauer der Füllung erreicht werden konnte. Für die wissenschaftliche Nachuntersuchung der Qualität von Füllungen müssen verschiedene Kriterien berücksichtigt werden. Einflüsse auf die Lebensdauer und Qualität der Füllung haben nicht nur das Material, sondern auch der Zahnarzt und der Patient (vgl. Jokstad et al., im Druck). So bestehen große Unterschiede in der Diagnose des Erneuerungsbedarfs von Füllungen (vgl. Bader und Shugars, 1995; Elderton, 1976; Maryniuk, 1990; Tveit und Espelid, 1992).

Die Vorteile von adhäsiven Füllungen werden meist in der Möglichkeit einer minimalinvasiven Versorgung gesehen, woraus langfristige Vorteile bezüglich der Lebensdauer und der Erhaltung des Zahnes abgeleitet werden (vgl. Tyas et al., im Druck). Die Evidenz für diese Behauptung ist allerdings noch recht spärlich. Veränderungen bezüglich der Indikationsstellung für die adhäsive direkte oder laborgefertigte Versorgung sind ebenfalls zu erwarten (vgl. Burke et al., 1991; Scheibenbogen et al., 1998).

Die klinische Evidenz von Vergleichen zwischen Amalgam und anderen Füllungsmaterialien muss jedoch auch von den Wünschen und Ansprüchen der Patienten ausgehen. Hier ist heute ein eindeutiger Trend zu ästhetischen Füllungsmaterialien zu sehen, und die Motivation dieser Patienten, die zahnfarbene Restaurationen wünschen, dürfte sicher nicht schlechter sein als die von den Patienten, die eine Standardversorgung wünschen. Die Problematik von Untersuchungen zur Langlebigkeit von Füllungsmaterialien liegt aber auch in der Durchführung der Studie. Meistens werden prospektiv-longitudinale Studien an Universitäten durchgeführt, die nicht den Gesetzmäßigkeiten und Zwängen der Praxis unterliegen. Retrospektive Untersuchungen in Praxen konnten jedoch zeigen, dass für Amalgamfüllungen zum Teil sehr ordentliche Werte gefunden wurden (vgl. Jokstad und Mjör, 1991). Andere Studien, berichten jedoch von einer recht kurzen Lebensdauer von Amalgam- und Komposit-Füllungen (vgl. Friedel, Hiller und Schmalz, 1994 und 1995).

Prospektive Studien mit neuen Füllungsmaterialien werden selten über längere Zeiträume durchgeführt. Dies ist neben dem Aufwand für solche Studien auch durch den häufigen Generationswechsel bei adhäsiven Füllungsmaterialen und Dentin-Bonding-Systemen begründet: Es kommen Hersteller mit verbesserten Materialien auf den Markt, so dass die alten Materialien uninteressant werden.

Die mittlere Lebensdauer von adhäsiven Restaurationen hat sich in den letzten Jahren erhöht (vgl. Abb. 7-4; Mjör, Jokstad und Qvist, 1990; Tyas et al., im Druck; Hickel, 1998; Bayne, 1992). Ob dies nun ein Trend ist, der durch die Verbesserung der Füllungsmaterialien bedingt ist oder aber durch eine andere Einstellung der Patienten und Zahnärzte mitverursacht wird, kann so nicht entschieden werden, da die Versuchsbedingungen unterschiedlich waren. Sehr wenig Evidenz ist derzeit über die ästhetische Zahnheilkunde verfügbar (vgl. Niederman et al., 1998)

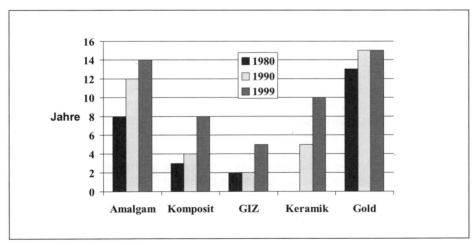

Abbildung 7-4: Lebensdauer von Restaurationen (modifiziert nach Bayne, 1992; Hickel, 1998; Tyas et al., im Druck)

7.5 Kosteneffektivität der Versorgung

Je nach der Kariesprävalenz und dem Kariesrisiko der Bevölkerung werden unterschiedliche Empfehlungen bezüglich der Notwendigkeit von Interventionen gegeben. So wurden in Schweden vor Jahren die regelmäßigen Fluoridspülungen in der Schule gestoppt, da der Kariesbefall so niedrig war, dass keine entsprechende Notwendigkeit und Kosteneffektivität (vgl. Sköld et al., 1998; Petersson, Netuschil und Brecx, im Druck) mehr gewährleistet waren. In der Schweiz wird die Verwendung der Fissurenversiegelung nicht mehr im großen Stil empfohlen, sondern nur noch für wenige Kinder mit sehr hohem Kariesrisiko. Der in Deutschland beobachtete Kariesrückgang der letzten Jahre ist nicht nur durch die häufigere Verwendung von Fluoriden begründet, sondern auch durch die seit 1992 von der GKV bezahlten Fissurenversiegelungen. Die Häufigkeit von Fissurenversiegelungen der Molaren von Kindern ist in den letzten Jahren z.T. auf über 60% gestiegen (vgl. Reich, 1996 und 1999), so dass hier die kariesanfälligste Fläche im Mund vor Karies geschützt wird.

Kosteneffektivität muss also im Einzelfall vom Zahnarzt für jeden Patienten entschieden werden. Die Kosteneffektivität bestimmter Interventionen für das Gesundheitssystem muss aufgrund des Kariesbefalls und des Kariesrisikos sowie der Versorgungsmöglichkeit beurteilt werden. Für die zahnärztliche Versorgung in Deutschland bedeutet dies, dass die Bewertungsmaßstäbe für die Vergütung zahnärztlicher Leistungen dringend überarbeitet werden müssen, um die Versorgung zu verbessern.

Das Problem der Kosteneffektivität zahnärztlicher Versorgung variiert natürlich in verschiedenen Ländern sehr stark, abhängig von den dort geltenden Abrechnungsbedingungen. Da aufgrund des wesentlich höheren Zeitaufwandes mit Kompositfüllungen und anderen adhäsiven Versorgungen auch höhere Kosten verbunden sind, deren Lebensdauer aber meistens eher geringer bewertet wird als die von Amalgamfüllungen, sind Amalgamfüllungen bei vergleichbaren Kavitäten als kostengünstiger einzustufen (vgl. Chadwick et al., 1999).

Nach einer Maßgabe der ADA muss eine neue Therapie eine mehr als 10%ige Verbesserung gegenüber der akzeptierten Standardtherapie aufweisen. Dies ist für die Kariestherapie und neue Füllungsmaterialien schwierig zu belegen, da sehr unterschiedliche Kriterien für die Bewertung des Erfolges angewandt werden.

In der Zahnerhaltung verwendete Erfolgskriterien sind:

– keine Karieszunahme,
– Erhaltung der Vitalität der Pulpa oder Erhaltung des Zahnes,
– Lebensdauer der Restauration.

Die Evidenz einer Maßnahme muss bezüglich der klinischen Signifikanz für jeden Patienten individuell vom Zahnarzt beurteilt werden. In Deutschland wie in anderen Industrieländern wird die Lebensdauer von Füllungen meist durch Zahnärzte im Sinne einer Therapieentscheidung mitbeeinflusst. Die Qualitätssicherung sollte verstärkt in die zahnärztlichen Aus- und Weiterbildung aufgenommen werden, da diesbezüglich Kriterien zur Entscheidungsoptimierung sehr fraglich sind (vgl. Maupomé, 1998). Es ist davon auszugehen, dass auch in Deutschland manche Füllungen unnötigerweise zu früh erneuert werden, die repariert werden oder auch durch Versiegelungsmaßnahmen noch länger in Funktion bleiben könnten. Hier sind neue Konzepte und Information durch Universitäten und Fortbildungsinstitute gefragt.

Es sollten auch im deutschen Gesundheitssystem für Zahnärzte Anreize zur kosteneffektiven Versorgung der Bevölkerung geschaffen werden, so dass die Effektivität in einem guten Verhältnis zum Aufwand steht.

Bei der Information des Patienten über die Auswahl von Füllungsmaterialien müssen diese Vor- und Nachteile dargestellt werden, so dass der Zahnarzt mit dem Patienten eine sinnvolle Auswahl treffen kann. Inwieweit die Kosten im Gesundheitssystem durch die evidenz-basierte Analyse reduziert werden, ist schwer vorhersehbar. Durch eine evidenz-basierte Zahnerhaltung sollten die Gefahr einer Übertherapie verringert und die individuelle Versorgung durch Verbesserungen in Diagnose und Intervention gesteigert werden.

Voraussetzung für diese positive Entwicklung ist aber die Implementierung der besten Evidenz in der Praxis. Hier hat die Wissenschaft die Aufgabe, die Evidenz so verständlich darzulegen, z. B. durch die Formulierung von Leitlinien, dass die Umsetzung in der Praxis möglichst einfach ist. Wissenschaftliche Studien über evidenz-basierte Therapievergleiche und die Erstellung von Leitlinien müssen über Drittmittelfinanzierung für die Wissenschaft durchführbar sein. Die Implementierung der Evidenz in der Praxis hängt neben der klaren Darstellung der Evidenz und der Begründung der Maßnahmen auch von der technischen und wirtschaftlichen Machbarkeit ab. Die zeitweise starke Zunahme von Versiegelungen der Molaren bei Kindern in Bayern (vgl. Reich, 1999) ist ein Beispiel, wie durch eine Veränderung der GKV-Richtlinien und Abrechnungsbedingungen eine sinnvolle Maßnahme schnell in der Praxis Verbreitung finden konnte.

7.6 Ausblick

Bisher ist deutschsprachige Literatur zur Evidenz in der Kariesprävention und -therapie nur sehr spärlich vorhanden. Hier ist die Wissenschaft gefordert, für die Produktion und Verbreitung dieser Evidenz zu sorgen. Um für die Praxis relevante Aussagen machen zu können, müssen umfassende

Analysen der Literatur durchgeführt werden, die auch Überlegungen bezüglich „klinischer zu statistischer" Signifikanz berücksichtigen (vgl. Rethman und Nunn, 1999). Durch Wissensvermittlung in der Fortbildung und der Ausbildung von Zahnmedizinern ist die Integration evidenz-basierter Maßnahmen in die Praxis zu ermöglichen. Die Implementierung der Evidenz setzt aber auch die wirtschaftlichen Grundlagen für deren Umsetzung voraus.

7 Evidence-based dentistry in caries therapy

Elmar Reich, Homburg/Saar

7.1 Preliminary note

The fundamentals of evidence-based medicine were described for the first time only in the last few years. EBM does not aim for a different kind of scientific basis, but it is defined by Sackett et al. (1996) as follows: "Evidence-based medicine is the conscientious, explicit, and judicious use of current best evidence in making decisions about the care of individual patients."

Evidence-based conservative dentistry could from this point of view be deemed to be the appropriate application of comprehensive diagnosis and intervention for the preservation of the patient's teeth and attachment apparatus (cf. McGuire & Nunn, 1996).

A recent study of adults in German dental practices (cf. Bauer & Huber, 1999) caused a stir because it revealed widely divergent treatment plans and costs for one and the same patient under different dentists. Similarly, the Readers Digest (cf. Eckenberger, 1997) reported on treatment plans drawn up by 50 American dentists at costs ranging between $500 and $30000.

Evidence-based conservative dentistry is expected to provide the following:

- individual care coupled with improved quality, durability, functionality and aesthetic appearance of the treated teeth,
- improvements in the dental health system, characterized by better quality and reduced costs.

The available evidence in the following three fields of conservative dentistry will now be examined:

- caries diagnosis,
- prevention,
- therapy.

7.2 Evidence in caries diagnosis

By far the largest number of scientific papers presented at the biggest dental-science conference, organized by the International Association for Dental Research (IADR) (cf. J Dent Res, 1999), were devoted to the fields of materials science and restorative therapy, followed way behind by studies on caries diagnosis and prevention. However, detection by probe or other aids is not the only available approach to the medical diagnosis of caries (cf. Reich, 1997; von Ohle & Reich, 1997; Lussi, 1998). The individual risk of caries should also be determined (cf. Reich, Lussi & Newbrun, 1999). Each patient's individual treatment needs can be determined on the basis of these findings (cf. Benn & Melzer, 1998; Edelstein, 1994; Berkey, Shay & Holm-Pedersen, 1996).

The sensitivity and specificity of different methods of caries diagnosis have been ascertained by complex studies (cf. Lussi et al., 1999; Verdonschot et al., 1999). Depending on caries location, visual and probe methods are found to have a sensitivity of only about 50%. Radiographic techniques yield only a slight improvement in average performance. Nor are other technical procedures, such as fibre-optic transillumination (FOTI), capable of appreciably improving the diagnosis. Better results are, however, obtained by laser-fluorescence techniques (cf. Lussi et al., 1999; Fig. 7-1) or electrical impedance measurement (ERM; cf. Verdonschot et al., 1999).

For approximal caries, radiographic techniques currently give the most reliable results, once the findings have been corrected for clinical misdiagnoses (cf. Verdonschot et al., 1999; Fig. 7-2). No substantial improvement was achieved by visual or probe examination or the use of FOTI. Initial results with laser fluorescence, however, suggest a promising potential at approximal surfaces (cf. Longbottom et al., 1999a; Eggertsson et al., 1999; Wagner, Longbottom & Pitts, 1999).

The gold standard for caries diagnosis is seen as the dentine demineralization or cavitation (cf. Ekstrand et al., 1998; Longbottom et al., 1999b). However, this gold standard calls for critical evaluation because it does not allow determination of the intervention requirement for incipient lesions, especially where prophylactic measures are still capable of stopping caries progression (cf. Pitts & Longbottom, 1995; Pine & Ten Bosch, 1996; Reich, 1997; von Ohle & Reich, 1997). Careful clinical diagnosis can already detect incipient enamel demineralization, which is eight times as frequent as caries-related cavities in the dentine of German 12-year-olds (cf. Schiffner & Reich, 1999). This means that the standard diagnosis based on the axiom "caries = cavity" no longer is clinically acceptable. Comprehensive medical diagnosis of caries is essential precisely in dental practices. The intervention requirement then breaks down into restoration, combined with prevention for carious cavities, and individual prophylactic measures where only incipient lesions are observable clinically or demineralization is revealed by

7.2 Evidence in caries diagnosis

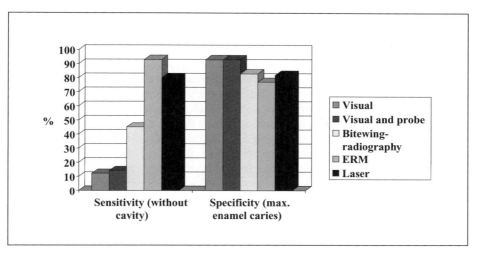

Figure 7-1: Sensitivity and specificity of different diagnostic methods for occlusal caries (cf. Lussi et al., 1999)

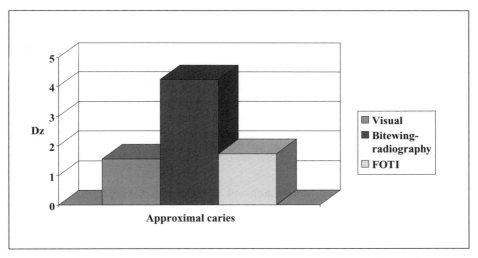

Figure 7-2: Average effectiveness (Dz) of different diagnostic techniques for approximal caries (cf. Verdonschot et al., 1999)

technical systems (cf. Pitts & Kidd, 1992; Pitts & Longbottom, 1995; Lussi, 1999; Netuschil, Dahmen & Reich, 1999).

Risk assessment for periodontal disease (cf. Page & Beck, 1997) and caries (cf. Reich, Lussi & Newbrun, 1999) is a new procedure to which relatively great uncertainty still attaches. However, the use of commercially available microbiological tests or saliva tests by themselves, without evaluation of clinical factors, does not permit a sufficiently precise estimate of the risk of pathology for the purpose of treatment planning.

The intervention requirement for preventive or invasive measures can thus be determined in practice after a comprehensive medical caries diagnosis. Since too many interventions would constitute overtreatment and hence be unnecessarily expensive, the requirement must be identified by a medical diagnosis. Preventive measures applied by the patient himself or herself, or undertaken professionally at the dental practice, are unlikely to have adverse effects. This is not the case, however, with invasive therapies (cf. Elderton & Mjör, 1992), where unnecessary fillings may result in consequential damage to the tooth or – owing to side-effects – the entire organism. Once caries has been diagnosed, little agreement is found to exist on the appropriate treatment (cf. Amer et al., 1998; Tveit, Espelid & Skodje, 1999).

An important problem still awaiting a satisfactory scientific solution is the diagnosis of secondary caries and identification of the replacement requirement for restorations (cf. Kidd, 1996; Mjör, 1981; Jokstad et al., in print). In industrialized nations with a properly functioning dental care system, restoration replacement accounts for a very high proportion – about 60% – of all restorative measures (cf. Chadwick et al., 1999). However, the life of a restoration is usually determined by the dentist, whose diagnosis establishes the need for its replacement (cf. Tveit & Espelid, 1992). Alternative options available today are cheaper and less invasive techniques such as the repair of restorations (cf. Ettinger, 1990; Mjör, 1993) or additional sealing measures.

7.3 Evidence in prevention

The effect of fluorides has recently been determined more precisely (cf. Ashley et al., 1999; CDA, 1999; ten Cate, 1999), with the following results:

- a dose/effect relationship exists between fluoride concentration and caries reduction;
- the frequency of tooth cleaning is positively correlated with caries reduction;
- rinsing with water after tooth cleaning adversely affects caries reduction;
- there is no definite correlation between toothpaste quantity and caries reduction.

A large number of studies have shown that fluorides do prevent caries. Nevertheless, the recommendations on their use differ (cf. WHO, 1994; CDA, 1994; CDA, 1999), and a number of reviews of the evidence on optimum fluoride application are nearing completion.

The Consensus Conference of the Canadian Dental Association (cf. CDA, 1999) came to the following conclusions on daily fluoride use (cf. Table 7-1, evidence levels as stated) (cf. Canadian Task Force, 1988):

Table 7-1: Consensus Conference of the Canadian Dental Association – conclusion on daily fluoride use

1. Fluoride has a predominantly topical effect.	Evidence level II-3
2. Water fluoridation is effective owing to its topical action.	Evidence level II
3. Fluoridated toothpaste is an effective means of topical application of fluorides.	Evidence level I
4. Swallowing more than the recommended daily dose of fluoride increases the risk of dental fluorosis.	Evidence level II-2
5. If topical fluorides – in particular, fluoride toothpaste or fluoridated drinking water – are not used in sufficient quantity, supplementary fluoride products in the form of rinses, chewing tablets or drops should be administered. The efficacy of these fluoride products: – is slight in the case of schoolchildren – has been studied only rarely in infants.	 Evidence level II-2 Evidence level II-3
6. Where the risk of caries is very high, the use of topical fluorides alone may not suffice to prevent caries. Supplementary fluoride use can have only a slight effect, and other measures, such as antimicrobial therapy and changes of diet, may be necessary.	Evidence level III

Source: CDA, 1999

As to diet, sugar-free chewing gums may also help in caries prophylaxis (cf. Imfeld, 1999).

Fissure sealing is an effective method of preventing occlusal caries, but the figures for its efficacy vary because they depend on caries prevalence, the risk of caries and also sealing material retention. The study by Mertz-Fairhurst et al. (1984) showed 50% caries reduction after seven years, with a retention rate of 66%. After 15 years (cf. Simonsen, 1991), caries or restorations were found in 31% of the originally sealed surfaces, compared with 83% for unsealed surfaces. A number of clinical studies have shown that sealing also has a significant preventive effect precisely in caries-susceptible children (cf. Straffon & Dennison, 1988). However, monitoring and where applicable resealing are necessary where sealing material has been lost from a surface. Yet according to Mitchell & Murray (1989), studies confirming the overall cost-effectiveness of sealing are still lacking. Precisely in Germany, where the legal health insurance scheme has been extended to cover sealing for children only in the last few years, this procedure substantially

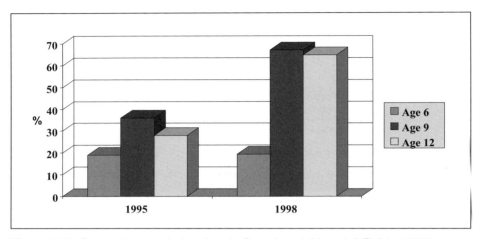

Figure 7-3: Percentage sealed molars in Bavarian children (cf. Reich, 1999)

accounts for the observed decline in caries (cf. Fig. 7-3; Reich, 1999; Schiffner & Reich, 1999). The retention period for both sealants and amalgam fillings in the molars of children aged between five and eight is, according to Mitchell & Murray (1989), only about two years, although this problem is no doubt specific to the treatment of children.

Other methods, such as the application of fluorides (cf. Stephen, 1995) or antibacterial products (cf. Petersson, Netuschil & Brecx, in print), may perfectly well be favourable in individual cases and adequate for preventing caries. However, this situation must be verified (by caries monitoring). The use of glass ionomer cements is also promising, according to Seppä & Forss (1991) and our own studies. For lasting prevention, inexpensive but effective techniques coupled with sealing based on individual risk criteria are appropriate (cf. Carvalho, Thylsturp & Ekstrand, 1992; Bader & Shugars, 1993). The value of oral health education in promoting dental health is generally considered questionable (cf. Kay & Locker, 1996). The provision of information on fluoride use has, however, been shown to be effective. Individual health education in the dental chair appears to be more effective than information imparted via the media.

7.4 Evidence in therapy

The principle of "complete" removal of carious dentine has been applied since the beginnings of scientific dentistry. Nevertheless, long-established concepts or dogmas should be questioned in the domain of therapy as elsewhere. The following fields may be analysed:

- caries therapy,
- indications for plastic filling materials,
- choice of filling or inlay/crown.

Whether consciously or unconsciously, the dogma of caries removal is not always observed in practice. In view of the difficulties of caries diagnosis ("hidden caries"), it may be assumed that up to 35% of carious fissures (cf. Weerheijm et al., 1990; Weerheijm, Groen & Poorterman, 1999; Ricketts et al., 1997) are sealed in spite of the presence of dentine caries. We now have a 10-year study (cf. Mertz-Fairhurst et al., 1998), conducted under clinically controlled conditions, in which dentine caries was either removed and the cavity treated with a conventional amalgam filling, or left, the cavity then being treated with a chemical-hardening composite and additional fissure sealing. A further group of amalgam fillings were additionally sealed. The results after 10 years showed that irreversible pulpitis had seldom arisen even where the caries had been left and sealed against bacteria. The failure rates for sealed composite fillings and classical amalgam fillings were comparable.

Owing to the large number of available materials and to patient demand for aesthetic fillings, it is not easy to decide which plastic filling material is appropriate in an individual case. According to the latest analyses, based on currently available evidence, amalgam is the longest-lasting and cheapest filling material (cf. Chadwick et al., 1999). Again, new restorative materials are often marketed without adequate subsequent clinical monitoring by scientific studies (cf. Roulet, 1997). Evaluation of 195 studies (cf. Chadwick et al., 1999) in which filling replacement criteria were specified and which took the form either of prospective longitudinal cohort studies or randomized clinical studies, showed that:

- amalgam appears more durable than composite;
- there were only slight differences between composite and ceramic inlays;
- amalgam fillings were more cost-effective than adhesive composite fillings or adhesive inlays.

A proviso here, however, is that the available clinical studies on composites differed from the amalgam studies in methodology and period of observation.

Another criticism levelled at many studies was that they often lacked objective parameters for determining quality and longevity. The criteria for replacement of restorations were usually not exactly defined, presumably with the consequence of reducing their service life, which was thus shorter than their potential life. A number of different criteria must be taken into account in the scientific monitoring of filling quality. Not only the material but also the dentist and the patient affect a filling's life and quality (cf. Jokstad et al., in print). Major differences thus exist in diagnosis of the replacement requirement for fillings (cf. Bader & Shugars, 1995; Elderton, 1976; Maryniuk, 1990; Tveit & Espelid, 1992).

Because invasiveness is minimized with adhesive fillings, they are thought to have long-term advantages in terms of longevity and tooth preservation (cf. Tyas et al., in print). However, the evidence for this assertion is still quite sparse. Changes in the indications for direct or laboratory-prepared adhesive restorations may also be expected (Burke et al., 1991; Scheibenbogen et al., 1998).

However, the clinical evidence on comparisons between amalgam and other filling materials must also take account of patient wishes and demands. In this connection, the trend today is for aesthetic filling materials to be used; the motivation of patients requiring tooth-coloured restorations must surely be rated no less highly than that of patients who want standard fillings. However, another problem with studies on the longevity of filling materials is the way they are conducted. They usually take the form of prospective longitudinal studies at universities, which are not subject to the fixed demands and constraints of a dental practice. Yet retrospective analyses from practices have in some cases yielded quite respectable values for amalgam fillings (cf. Jokstad & Mjör, 1991). Other studies, conversely, report that the life of amalgam and composite restorations is quite short (cf. Friedel, Hiller & Schmalz, 1994 and 1995).

Prospective studies of new filling materials are seldom conducted over extended periods. This is due not only to the complexity and expense of such studies but also to the frequent succession of generations of adhesive filling materials and dentine bonding systems: manufacturers market improved materials, so that the old ones become unattractive.

The average life of adhesive restorations has increased in recent years (cf. Fig. 7-4; Mjör, Jokstad & Qvist, 1990; Tyas et al., in print; Hickel, 1998; Bayne, 1992). Owing to variable experimental conditions, it is impossible to decide whether this trend is due to improved filling materials or whether changed attitudes on the part of patients and dentists are a contributory factor. Very little evidence is currently available on aesthetic dentistry (cf. Niederman et al., 1998).

7.5 Cost-effectiveness of treatment

Depending on caries prevalence and the caries risk in the population, recommendations on the need for intervention differ. For example, regular fluoride rinses in school were halted in Sweden many years ago because caries levels were so low that this measure was no longer necessary or cost-effective (cf. Sköld et al., 1998; Petersson, Netuschil & Brecx, in print). Fissure sealing is no longer recommended for large-scale application in

7.5 Cost-effectiveness of treatment

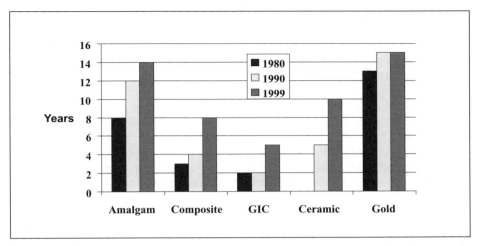

Figure 7-4: Longevity of restorations (cf. Bayne, 1992; Hickel, 1998; Tyas et al., in print [modified])

Switzerland, but only in a small number of children with a very high caries risk. The decline in caries observed in Germany in the last few years is due not only to the more frequent use of fluorides but also to the fact that the legal health insurance scheme has paid for fissure sealing since 1992. The frequency of fissure sealing in children's molars has increased in some cases to over 60% in the last few years (cf. Reich, 1996 and 1999), providing protection for the mouth's most caries-susceptible surface.

Cost-effectiveness must therefore be a matter for individual decision-making by the dentist for each patient. The cost-effectiveness of specific interventions from the point of view of the health system must be assessed on the basis of caries prevalence and risk and of treatment capacity. As regards dental care in Germany, this means that an urgent review of the assessment criteria for the remuneration of dental services is necessary in order to improve care.

Of course, the problem of the cost-effectiveness of dental care varies substantially from country to country in accordance with the applicable payment conditions. Composite restorations and other adhesive treatments are more time-consuming and therefore more expensive, and are also generally regarded as less durable than amalgam fillings, so that the latter must be regarded as less expensive overall for comparable cavities (cf. Chadwick et al., 1999).

According to a criterion adopted by the ADA, a new treatment must yield an improvement of more than 10% over the accepted standard therapy. Such proof is difficult to come by in the case of caries therapy and new filling materials, as widely differing criteria of success are applied.

The following criteria of success are used in conservative dentistry:

- no increase in caries,
- retention of pulp vitality or preservation of the tooth,
- longevity of restoration.

The evidence for a measure must be assessed by the dentist individually in terms of its clinical significance for each patient. In Germany as in other industrialized countries, filling life is usually partly determined by the dentist as a therapeutic decision. Quality assurance should play an increased part in dental education and continuing education, as the relevant criteria for the optimization of decision-making are highly questionable (cf. Maupomé, 1998). There is reason to believe that in Germany as elsewhere, some fillings are replaced unnecessarily early although they could have been repaired or kept operational for a longer period by sealing measures. On this point, new concepts and information are needed from our universities and continuing-education institutions.

Incentives to optimize the cost-effective care of the population like those existing in some other countries should also be introduced for dentists in the German health system.

Where patients are given information to help in the choice of filling materials, the relevant advantages and disadvantages must be explained, so that dentist and patient can together make a reasoned choice. It is difficult to predict the extent to which costs in the health system may be reduced by evidence-based analysis. Evidence-based tooth conservation may be expected to reduce the risk of overtreatment and enhance individual care through improvements in diagnosis and intervention.

However, such a positive trend is conditional upon the implementation of best evidence in the dental practice. Here science has the task of presenting the evidence in understandable form – e.g. by the formulation of guidelines – in such a way as to facilitate its transposition into practice. External funding is required for science so as to permit scientific evidence-based comparative therapy studies and the compilation of guidelines. Practical implementation depends not only on clear presentation of the evidence for and justification of measures but also on technical and economic feasibility. The big increase in children's molar sealing in Bavaria over a given period (cf. Reich, 1999) is an example of how a change in the legal health insurance scheme directives and payment conditions allowed the rapid dissemination of a desirable measure in practice.

7.6 Outlook

The German-language literature on evidence in caries prevention and therapy is as yet sparse. It is up to the scientific world to produce and disseminate this evidence. If relevant results are to be made available to dental practitioners, comprehensive literature analyses, allowing also for considerations of "clinical versus statistical" significance, must be conducted (cf. Rethman & Nunn, 1999). The integration of evidence-based measures into practice must be facilitated by imparting the relevant knowledge in dental education and continuing education. However, evidence implementation is conditional upon the existence of the appropriate economic basis.

7.7 Literatur/References

Amer, M. E., Omer, O. E., Bergquist, J., Elderton, R. J., Claffey, N.: Investigation of the operative response of a group of general dental practitioners to varying extents of proximal caries. Eur J Dent Educ 2 (1998), 65–68

Ashley, P. F., Attrill, D. C., Ellwood, R. P., Worthington, H. v., Davies, R. M.: Toothbrushing habits and caries experience. Caries Res 33 (1999), 401–402

Bader, J. D., Shugars, D. A.: Variation in dentists clinical decisions. J Public Health Dent 55 (1995), 181–188

Bader, J. D., Shugars, D. A.: Need for change in standards of caries diagnosis epidemiology and health services research perspective. J Dent Education 57 (1993), 415–421

Bauer, J., Huber, H.: Markttransparenz beim Zahnarzt. Institut für angewandte Verbraucherforschung e.V./Wissenschaftliches Institut der AOK, Bonn (1999)

Bayne, S. C.: Dental composites/glass ionomers: clinical reports. Adv Dent Res 6 (1992), 65–77

Benn, D. K., Melzer, M.: Will modern caries management reduce restorations in dental practice? J Am Coll Dent 63 (1998), 39–44

Berkey, D. B., Shay, K., Holm-Pedersen, P.: Clinical decision-making for the elderly dental patient. Textbook of Gen Dent (1996), 319–337

Burke, F. J. T., Watts, D. C., Wilson, N. H. F., Wilson, M. A.: Current status and rationale for composite inlays and onlays. British Dent J 6 (1991), 269–273

Canadian Task Force under periodic health examination: The periodic health examination: Can Med Assoc J, 138 (1988), 618–626

Carvalho, J. C., Thylstrup, A., Ekstrand, K. R.: Results after 3 years of non-operative occlusal caries treatment of erupting permanent first molars. Community Dent Oral Epidemiol 20 (1992), 187–192

CDA (Canadian Dental Association): Report of the canadian workshop on the evaluation of current recommendations concerning fluorides (1992). Community Dent Oral Epidemiol 22 (1994), 133–186

CDA (Canadian Dental Association): Proceedings of the Consensus Conference of the Canadian Dental Association (1997): Appropriate use of fluoride supplements for the prevention of dental caries. Community Dent Oral Epidemiol 27 (1999), 27–83

Chadwick, B. L., Dummer, P. M. H., Dunstan, F. D., Gilmour, A. S. M., Jones, R. J., Phillips, C. J., Rees, J., Richmond, S., Stevens, J., Treasure, T. E.: What type of filling? Best practice in dental restorations. Quality in Health Care 8 (1999), 202–207

Eckenberg: Readers Digest, März 1997, USA

Edelstein, B. L.: The medical management of dental caries. J Am Dent Assoc 125 (1994), 31–39

Eggertsson, H., Analoui, M., van der Veen, M. H., González-Cabezas, C., Eckert, G. J., Stookey, G. K.: Detection of early interproximal caries in vitro using laser fluorescence, dye-enhanced laser fluorescence and direct visual examination. Caries Res 33 (1999), 227–233

7.7 Literatur/References

Ekstrand, K. R., Ricketts, D. N. J., Kidd, E. A. M., Qvist, V., Schou, S.: Detection, diagnosing, monitoring and logical treatment of occlusal caries in relation to lesion activity and severity: An in vivo examination with histological validation. Caries Res 32 (1998), 247–254

Elderton, R. J.: The causes of failure of restorations: A literature review. J Dent 6 (1976), 257–262

Elderton, R. J., Mjör, I. A.: Changing scene in cariology and operative dentistry. Int Dent J 42 (1992), 165–169

Ettinger, R.: Restoring the aging dentition: repair or replacement? Int Dent J 40 (1990), 275–282

Friedel, K. H., Hiller, K. A., Schmalz, G.: Placement and replacement of amalgam restorations in Germany. Oper Dent 19 (1994), 228–232

Friedel, K. H., Hiller, K. A., Schmalz, G.: Placement and replacement of composite restorations in Germany. Oper Dent 20 (1995), 34–37

Hickel, R.: Longevity of restorative materials. Vortrag IADR Symposium Nizza 1998

Imfeld, T.: Chewing gum – facts and fiction: A review of gum-chewing and oral health. Crit Rev Oral Biol Med 3 (1999), 405–419

Jokstad, A., Mjör, I. A.: Analyses of long-term clinical behavior of class-II amalgam restorations. Acta Odontol Scand 49 (1991), 47–63

Jokstad, A., Osborne, J., Blunck, U., Tyas, M., van Noort, R.: Quality of restorations. Int Dent J (im Druck/in print)

Journal of Dental Research 78, Special Issue (IADR-Abstracts), 1999

Kay, E. J., Locker, D.: Is dental health education effective? A systematic review of current evidence. Commun Dent Oral Epidemiol 24 (1996), 231–235

Kidd, E. A. M.: Diagnosis of secondary caries. In: Stookey G. K. (Hrsg.): Early detection of dental caries. Indianapolis, 1996, 156–163

Longbottom, C., Wagner, M., Pitts, N. B., Lussi, A.: Simulated in vivo comparison of bitewing radiography and DIAGNOdent for approximal caries detection. Caries Res 33 (1999a), Abstract 52, 298

Longbottom, C., Pitts, N. B., Lussi, A., Reich, E.: Histological validation of in vivo measurements using the DIAGNOdent device: A Three-Centre Study. Caries Res 33 (1999b), Abstract 58, 300

Lussi, A.: Methoden zur Diagnose und Verlaufsdiagnose der Karies. Dtsch Zahnärztl. Z 53 (1998), 175

Lussi, A., Imwinkelried, S., Pitts, N. B., Longbottom, C., Reich, E.: Performance and reproducibility of a laser fluorescence system for detection of occlusal caries in vitro. Caries Res 33 (1999), 261–266

Lussi, A.: Methoden zur Diagnose und Verlaufsdiagnose der Karies. Oralprophylaxe 21 (1999), 67–75

Maryniuk, G.: Practice variation: learned and socioeconomic factors. Advances in Dental Research 4 (1990), 19–24

Maupomé, G.: A comparison of senior dental students and normative standards with regard to caries assessment and treatment decisions to restore occlusal surfaces of permanent teeth. J Prosthetic Dent 76 (1998), 596–603

McGuire, M. K., Nunn, M. E.: Prognosis versus actual outcome. II. The effectiveness of clinical parameters in developing an accurate prognosis. J Periodontol 7 (1996), 658–674

Mertz-Fairhurst, E. J., Fairhurst, C. W., Williams, J. E., Della-Ciustiana, V. E., Brooks, J. D.: A comparative clinical study of two pit and fissure sealants: 7-year results in Augusta, GA. J Am Dent Assoc 109 (1984), 252–255

Mertz-Fairhurst, E. J., Curtis, J. W., Ergle, J. W., Rueggeberg, F. A., Adair, S. M.: Ultraconservative and cariostatic sealed restorations: results at year 10. J Am Dent Assoc 129 (1998), 55–66

Mitchell, L., Murray, J. J.: Fissure sealants: a critique of their cost-effectiveness. Community Dent Oral Epidemiol 17 (1989), 19–23

Mjör, I. A.: Placement and replacement of restorations. Oper Dent 6 (1981), 49–54

Mjör, I. A.: Long term cost of restorative therapy using different materials. Scand J Dent Res 100 (1992), 60–65

Mjör, I. A.: Repair versus replacement of failed restorations. Int Dent J 43 (1993), 466–472

Mjör, I. A., Jokstad A., Qvist, V.: Longevity of posterior restorations. Int Dent J 40 (1990), 11–17

Netuschil, L., Dahmen, F., Reich, E.: Efficacy of fluoride preparations on early carious lesions. Caries Res 33 (1999), Abstract 67

Niederman, R., Ferguson, M., Urdaneta, R., Badovinac, R., Christie, D., Tantraphol, M., Rasool, F.: Evidence-Based Esthetic Dentistry. J Esthetic Dent 10 (1998), 229–234

Page, R. C., Beck, J. D.: Risk assessment for periodontal diseases. Int Dent J 47 (1997), 61–87

Petersson, L., Netuschil, L., Brecx, M.: Mouthrinses against caries. Int Dent J (im Druck/in print)

Pine, C. M., ten Bosch, J. J.: Dynamics of and diagnostic methods for detecting small carious lesions. Caries Res 30 (1996), 381–388

Pitts, N. B., Kidd, E. A. M.: Some of the factors to be considered in the prescription and timing of bitewing radiography in the diagnosis and management of dental caries. J Dent 20 (1992), 74–84

Pitts, N. B., Longbottom, C.: Preventive Care (PCA) Operative Care Advised (OCA) – categorising caries by the management option. Community Dent Oral Epidemiol 23 (1995), 55–59

Reich, E.: Mundgesundheitszustand bayerischer Grundschüler. LAGZ München 1996

Reich, E.: Moderne Methoden der Kariesdiagnostik bestimmen die Therapieentscheidung. Zahnärztl Mitt 88 (1997), 1228–1235

Reich, E., Lussi, A., Newbrun, E.: Caries-risk assessment. Int Dent J 49 (1999), 15–26

Reich, E.: Zahngesundheit bayerischer Schulkinder 1998/99. LAGZ München 1999

Rethman, M. P., Nunn, M. E.: Clinical versus statistical significance. J Periodontol 6 (1999), 700–702

Ricketts, D., Kidd, E., Weerheijm, K., de Soet, H.: Hidden caries: What is it? Does it exist? Does it matter? Int Dent J 47 (1997), 259–265

Roulet, J. F.: Benefits and disadvantages of tooth-coloured alternatives to amalgam. J Dent 1997, 459–473

Sackett, D. L., Rosenberg, W. M., Gray, J. A., Haynes, R. B., Richardson, W. S.: Evidence based medicine: what it is and what it isn't. BMJ 312 (1996), 71–72

Scheibenbogen, A., Manhart, J., Kunzelmann, K. H., Hickel, R.: One-year clinical evaluation of composite and ceramic inlays in posterior teeth. J Prosthetic Dent 80 (1998), 410–416

Schiffner, U., Reich, E.: Karies/Füllungen bei den Jugendlichen. In: Dritte Deutsche Mundgesundheitsstudie (DMS III). Institut der Deutschen Zahnärzte (Hrsg.). Köln 1999, 201–230

Seppä, L., Forss, H.: Resistance of occlusal fissures to demineralization after loss of glass ionomer sealants in vitro. Pediatric Dent 13 (1991), 39–42

Simonsen, R. J.: Retention and effectiveness of dental sealant after 15 years. J Am Dent Assoc 122 (1991), 34–42

Sköld, U. M., Lindvall, A. M., Rasmusson, C. G., Birkhed, D., Klock, B.: Caries incidence in adolescence after cessation of weekly fluoride rinsing. J Dent Res 77 (1998), Abstract Nr. 67

Stephen, K. W.: The value of anti-caries and anti-plaque dentifrices at a community level. Adv Dent Res 2 (1995), 127

Straffon, L. H., Dennison, J. B.: Clinical evaluation comparing sealant and amalgam after 7 years: final report. J Am Dent Assoc 177 (1988), 751–755

ten Cate, R.: Vortrag "Fluoridwirkung" ADF Tagung 1999

Tveit, A., Espelid, I.: Class II amalgam interobserver variation in replacement decisions and diagnosis of caries and crevice. Int Dent J 42 (1992), 12–18

Tveit, A. B., Espelid, I., Skodje, F.: Restorative treatment decisions on approximal caries in Norway. Int Dent J 49 (1999), 165–172

Tyas, M. J., Anusavice, K. J., Frencken, J. E., Mount, G. J.: Minimal intervention dentistry – a review. Int Dent J (im Druck/in print)

Verdonschot, E. H., Angmar-Mansson, B., ten Bosch, J. J., Deery, C. H., Huysmans, M. C. D. N. J. M., Pitts, N. B., Waller, E.: Developments in caries diagnosis and their relationship to treatment decisions and quality of care. Caries Res 33 (1999), 32–40

von Ohle, C., Reich, E.: Moderne Kariestherapie. Diagnostik und Therapieplanung. Zahnarzt Magazin 1 (1997), 20

Wagner, M., Longbottom, C., Pitts, N. B.: An in vitro comparison of a laser device with bitewing radiography for approximal caries detection. Caries Res 33 (1999), Abstract 53, 298

Weerheijm, K. L., de Soet, J. J., de Graaff, J., van Amerongen, W. E.: Occlusal hidden caries: A bacteriological profile. J Dent Child (1990), 428–432

Weerheijm, K. L., Groen, H. J., Poorterman, J. H. G.: Clinically undetected occlusal dentine caries in 1987 and 1993 in 17-year-old Dutch adolescents. Caries Res 33 (1999), Abstract 21, 288

WHO: Fluorides and oral health, Technical Report Series 846, Genf 1994

8 Evidenz-basierte Konzepte in der parodontologischen Praxis

Jörg Meyle, Gießen

8.1 Einleitung

Evidenz-basierte Medizin (EBM) ist in der fachlichen und nicht fachlichen Öffentlichkeit zu einem geflügelten Wort geworden. EBM ist keine neue Erfindung, sondern schon seit dem 19. Jahrhundert bekannt, wurde aber durch die Publikationen der englischen Gruppe um Sackett neu aufgegriffen und durch Gründung der Cochrane Collaboration institutionalisiert (vgl. Richards, Lawrence und Sackett, 1997; Sackett, 1998). Jeder verantwortungsbewusste Arzt wird sich in seiner Diagnostik und Therapie an den anerkannten Regeln der Kunst, also dem lex artis orientieren, ansonsten könnte ihm der Vorwurf der Quacksalberei gemacht werden. Nichts anderes will evidenz-basierte Medizin, die auf wissenschaftliche Evidenz, d. h. auf soliden wissenschaftlichen Erkenntnissen, beruht.

In der Parodontologie gibt es durch eine große Anzahl wissenschaftlicher Vergleichsstudien für verschiedene therapeutische Bereiche eine solide wissenschaftliche Evidenz. Das Problem in Deutschland besteht darin, dass der z. Z. noch gültige Behandlungsvertrag in der vertragszahnärztlichen Versorgung eine zahnärztliche Diagnostik und Therapie aufbauend auf der aktuellen wissenschaftlichen Evidenz (vgl. Tab. 8-1) nicht zulässt. Wesentliche Abschnitte der parodontologischen Behandlung (Initialtherapie, unterstützende PAR-Therapie = Recall) sind bis heute nicht Bestandteil des Vertrages. Außerdem erfolgt keine klare Differenzierung der verschiedenen therapeutischen Maßnahmen, d.h. gemäss dem bestehenden Vertrag ist es möglich, Behandlungen durchzuführen und abzurechnen, von denen wir heute wissen, dass sie in dieser Form dem Patienten eher schaden als nützen.

8.2 Diagnostik und Initialtherapie

Da es sich bei der marginalen Parodontitis um eine ortsspezifische Erkrankung handelt, ist eine gründliche Untersuchung jedes einzelnen Zahnes an mehreren Stellen notwendig, um sich über Schwere und Ausdehnung Gewissheit zu verschaffen. Selbst bei einer Sondierung an 6 Stellen/Zahn wird

Tabelle 8-1: Vereinfachtes Schema des Behandlungsablaufes bei adulter Parodontitis im Vergleich zum bestehenden PAR-Vertrag

Behandlungsabschnitt	Behandlungsabschnitte in der GKV
Screeningbefund	–
Professionelle Zahnreinigung (Initialtherapie Phase I)	nicht Bestandteil des Vertrages (über Krankenschein abzurechnen)
Spezielle parodontologische Diagnostik	Untersuchung im Rahmen des PAR-Antrages
Wurzeloberflächenreinigung (Deep Scaling, Initialtherapie Phase II)	–
Zwischenbefundung	–
Korrektive/chirurgische Therapie	Maßnahmen nicht differenziert
Abschlussbefund	–
Unterstützende Therapie	–

nur ein Bruchteil (ca. 12%) des gesamten linearen Attachments erfasst. Die Messung der Sondierungstiefen an 2 bzw. 4 Stellen bildet keine sichere diagnostische Grundlage für die therapeutische Planung (vgl. Haffajee und Socransky, 1986).

Die Bedeutung der gründlichen und mehrfachen Mundhygieneinstruktion für den Erfolg der Lokaltherapie hat die Vergleichsstudie von Nyman, Lindhe und Rosling (1977) klar gezeigt. Wird nur eine einmalige Mundhygieneinstruktion vorgenommen, kommt es innerhalb des 1. Jahres zu einem Rezidiv des Plaquebefalls und der gingivalen Entzündung. Unter diesen Umständen sind alle weiterführenden Behandlungsmaßnahmen gleich wirkungslos. Die mehrfache gründliche Mundhygieneinstruktion und Objektivierung der Belagbildung unter Zuhilfenahme eines entsprechenden Indexsystems ist eine unabdingbare Voraussetzung für eine erfolgreiche Lokalbehandlung.

Bei aggressiven Formen der Parodontitis ist zusätzlich eine mikrobiologische Diagnostik sinnvoll, da durch hohe Anteile von A. actinomycetem comitans, P. gingivalis und B. forsythus in der subgingivalen Plaque der Erfolg der mechanischen Therapie fraglich ist. Es besteht internationaler Konsens, dass es sich bei diesen Keimen um Oralpathogene handelt (vgl. Zambon, 1996).

Außer der Beseitigung der supragingivalen Beläge und des Zahnsteins ist eine sorgfältige Reinigung aller erkrankten subgingivalen Wurzeloberflächen erforderlich, um die körpereigenen Heilungsprozesse soweit zu unterstüt-

Tabelle 8-2: Auswahl klinischer Vergleichsstudien[1] zur Effizienz der subgingivalen Wurzeloberflächenreinigung (Deep Scaling)				
Autor	Jahr	Art	Dauer (Monate)	Patienten (n)
Hill	1981	RCT	24	90
Pihlstrom	1981	RCT	6/48	17
Nordland	1987	Kohorten	24	19
Becker	1988	RCT	12	16
Kaldahl	1988	RCT	3	82
Loos	1989	Kohorten	24	12

[1] Insgesamt ca. 30 relevante Studien zu diesem Thema (Quelle: Ann Periodontol 1 [1996], S. 443–490)

zen, dass eine Ausheilung stattfinden kann. Die Effizienz der als Wurzeloberflächenreinigung (Deep scaling, Root planing) bezeichneten Maßnahme wurde von zahlreichen Autoren in randomisierten klinischen Vergleichsstudien (RCT) dokumentiert (vgl. Tab. 8-2).

Diese Untersuchungen zeigten, dass eine sorgfältige subgingivale Reinigung ausreicht, um ein ähnlich gutes Behandlungsergebnis zu erzielen, wie es in der Kombination mit chirurgischen Methoden möglich ist (vgl. Pihlstrom, Ortiz und McHugh, 1981). Es ist bekannt, dass selbst bei anfangs sehr tiefen Taschen mit Hilfe dieser Maßnahme eine Restsondierungstiefe von 4 mm erzielt werden kann (vgl. Knowles et al., 1979; Baderstein, Nilvéus und Egelberg, 1981; 1984a; 1984b; 1985a; 1985b; 1985c; 1985d; 1987).

An diesen Behandlungsabschnitt schließt sich die Zwischenbewertung bzw. Reevaluation an, in der alle Zähne erneut gründlich klinisch untersucht werden, um nach blutenden Resttaschen zu fahnden.

8.3 Weiterführende (chirurgische) Therapie

Sofern sich bei der Untersuchung zeigt, dass noch infizierte Resttaschen vorhanden sind oder eine Furkationsbeteiligung vorliegt, muss eine weiterführende PAR-Behandlung geplant werden. Mit Hilfe von chirurgischen Methoden werden die restlichen bakteriellen Auflagerungen und das Granulationsgewebe beseitigt und durch korrektive Maßnahmen entweder eine Regeneration des verloren gegangenen Halteapparates eingeleitet bzw. die Hygienefähigkeit des Gebisses weiter verbessert.

Für die weiterführende (chirurgische Parodontaltherapie) steht heute eine Reihe von verschiedenen Methoden zur Verfügung (vgl. Tab. 8-3). Bei tiefen Resttaschen hat die Meta-Analyse von Antczak-Bouckoms et al. (1993) ergeben, dass dort durch chirurgische Maßnahmen eine weitere Reduktion der Sondierungstiefe möglich ist, wohingegen bei flachen Taschen mit einem zusätzlichen Attachmentverlust gerechnet werden muss (vgl. Antczak-Bouckoms, 1993; Antczak-Bouckoms et al., 1993).

Verschiedene Vergleichsstudien belegen den Vorteil der regenerativen Behandlung (GTR), wobei aber in Abhängigkeit von der Defektmorphologie bzw. des beteiligten Zahnes die Erfolgsaussichten unterschiedlich groß sind (vgl. Laurell und Gottlow, 1998). So konnte in der Arbeit von Proestakis et al. (1992) kein eindeutiger Unterschied zwischen den regenerativ behandelten Stellen und den konventionell therapierten Zähnen beobachtet werden. Klare Vorteile zu Gunsten der regenerativen Behandlung ergaben sich bei der Therapie von Furkationsdefekten Grad II im Unterkiefer bzw. Furkationsdefekten Grad II an den Bukkalflächen der oberen Molaren (vgl. Pontoriero und Lindhe, 1995; Pontoriero et al., 1987; 1988; 1989).

Für den Langzeiterfolg der Gesamttherapie ist die regelmäßige Nachsorge nach Abschluss der korrektiven Behandlungsmaßnahmen von größter Bedeutung. Seit über 20 Jahren ist bekannt, dass bei einem regelmäßigen Recall (im Abstand von drei bis sechs Monaten) ein weiterer Zahnverlust über einen Zeitraum von zwei Jahrzehnten (!) vermieden werden kann, d. h. in Abhängigkeit von der Regelmäßigkeit der Nachsorge und der Mitarbeit des Patienten konnten über 90% aller erkrankten Zähne erhalten werden (vgl. Axelsson und Lindhe, 1981a; 1981b; Axelsson, Lindhe und Nyström,

Tabelle 8-3: Verfahren der Parodontalchirurgie zur Behandlung von entzündungsbedingten Defekten	
1. Resektive Verfahren zur Taschenelimination, -reduktion	apikaler Verschiebelappen bzw. apikal reponierter Lappen mit/ohne – Knochenresektion – distale Keilexzision Gingivektomie (extern, intern) Zugangslappen (modifizierter Widman-Lappen)
2. Regenerative Verfahren	regenerative Therapie (GTR) unter Verwendung von – Transplantaten – Implantaten (Membranen) – Wachstumsproteinen
3. Furkationstherapie	Tunnelierung Hemisektion, Radektomie

1991; Hirschfeld und Wasserman, 1978; McFall, 1982). In der Vergleichsstudie von Axelsson und Lindhe (1981a) wurde nachgewiesen, dass ohne Nachsorge ein frühzeitiges Erkrankungsrezidiv auftritt, das von einem weiteren Attachmentverlust begleitet wird.

8.4 Zusammenfassung

In den letzten Jahren wurde durch groß angelegte Studien in den Vereinigten Staaten belegt, dass die marginale Parodontitis Auswirkungen auf den allgemeinen Gesundheitszustand hat und u. a. das Risiko für eine Frühgeburt bzw. die Geburt eines untergewichtigen Kindes bei Schwangeren mit schwerer generalisierter Parodontitis bis zu sechsmal höher ist. Ebenso gilt es heute als gesichert, dass das Risiko für Herzinfarkt und Herz-Kreislauferkrankungen (u. a. Schlaganfall) durch eine marginale Parodontitis zunimmt (vgl. Beck et al., 1996; Beck et al., 1998; Offenbacher et al., 1996; 1998; Page et al., 1997; Salvi et al., 1997).

Sofern wissenschaftliche Evidenz die Grundlage unserer praktischen Tätigkeit sein soll, bedeutet das für die Parodontologie in der gesetzlichen Krankenversicherung (GKV) ein radikales Umdenken und die Einführung einer längst überfälligen Reform, die trotz jahrelanger Interventionen von Seiten der wissenschaftlichen Fachgesellschaft von den politisch Verantwortlichen immer wieder verschleppt wurde.

Dies allein wird nicht ausreichen, da gleichzeitig eine Verschiebung der Tätigkeitsschwerpunkte in der zahnärztlichen Praxis erfolgen muss. Die bisherige Dominanz der restaurativen Maßnahmen sollte zu Gunsten der Frühdiagnostik, Prävention und Erhaltung aufgegeben werden.

Dafür werden die Zahnärzte bis heute nicht ausgebildet. Im Zahnmedizinstudium, dessen Konzept im Wesentlichen auf den Erkenntnissen der 70er-Jahre (!) beruht, dominieren weiterhin restaurative Maßnahmen. Präventionsorientierte Fächer, wie die Parodontologie, haben nur einen unbedeutenden, nicht klar definierten Anteil am Gesamtcurriculum. Gerade die subgingivale Reinigung der infizierten Wurzeloberflächen (Deep Scaling), deren Effizienz nicht hoch genug eingeschätzt werden kann, erfordert aufgrund der anspruchsvollen Technik eine intensive Schulung. Eine Reform des Studiums würde mittelfristig zu einer deutlichen Verschiebung der Schwerpunkte in der zahnärztlichen Praxis und zu einem noch besseren Gesundheitszustand unserer Bevölkerung beitragen.

Eine detaillierte Übersicht über die wissenschaftliche Evidenz in unserem Fachgebiet würde den Rahmen dieses Beitrages sprengen. Eine Reihe von exzellenten Übersichten wurde dazu in den letzten Jahren veröffentlicht: insbesondere sei an dieser Stelle auf die Zusammenfassung des letzten World Workshops on Clinical Periodontics und die im Quintessenz-Verlag veröffentlichten Berichte der Europäischen Workshops verwiesen. Darüber hinaus werden in der Zeitschrift „Periodontology 2000" laufend aktuelle Literaturübersichten zu einzelnen Themen publiziert.

8 Evidence-based approaches to periodontal practice

Jörg Meyle, Gießen

8.1 Introduction

Evidence-based medicine (EBM) has become a set phrase in specialist and non-specialist circles alike. EBM is not a new invention but has been known since the nineteenth century; however, it gained renewed currency through the publications of the British group around Sackett and was institutionalized by the establishment of the Cochrane Collaboration (cf. Richards, Lawrence & Sackett, 1997; Sackett, 1998). Every responsible doctor will observe the accepted rules of his art – the lex artis – in his diagnosis and therapy if he is not to lay himself open to charges of quackery. Evidence-based medicine, based as it is on scientific evidence – i.e. on a solid foundation of scientific knowledge – has no other aim than to assist him in this regard.

In the field of periodontology the large number of comparative scientific studies existing in various therapeutic spheres offer a firm basis of scientific evidence. The problem in Germany is that the current treatment contract for dentists providing care within the legal health insurance fund system does not permit a dental diagnosis and therapy based on current scientific evidence (see Table 8-1). Important aspects of periodontal treatment (initial therapy and supportive periodontal care – i.e. recall) are even now not included in the contract. Furthermore, the various therapeutic measures are not clearly distinguished – that is to say, the present contract allows dentists to undertake and charge for forms of treatment which, as we now know, are more likely to harm than to benefit the patient.

8.2 Diagnosis and initial therapy

Since periodontitis is a site-specific disease, a thorough examination of each individual tooth at several different measuring points is necessary to be certain about the severity and extent of the defects. Even probing six points per tooth covers only a fraction (approximately 12%) of the entire linear attachment. Measurement of probing depth at two or four points does not afford a reliable diagnostic base for treatment planning (cf. Haffajee & Socransky, 1986).

Table 8-1: Simplified breakdown of treatment sequence for adult periodontitis vs existing periodontology contract

Stage of treatment	Periodontal treatment under the German legal health insurance scheme
Screening	–
Professional tooth cleaning (initial therapy Phase I)	Not covered by contract (to be charged by health insurance certificate)
Specific periodontal diagnosis	Examination under the system of application to the health insurance fund for periodontal treatment
Root surface cleaning (deep scaling, initial therapy Phase II)	–
Interim findings	–
Corrective or surgical therapy	Measures not distinguished
Final findings	–
Supporting therapy	–

The importance of thorough, repeated oral hygiene instructions for the success of local therapy was clearly demonstrated by the comparative study of Nyman, Lindhe & Rosling (1977). If oral hygiene instruction is given only once, plaque and gingival inflammation return within one year. In these circumstances, any further treatment measures are ineffective from the outset. Repeated thorough oral hygiene instruction and meticulous recording of plaque formation by an appropriate indexing system are essential preconditions for successful local treatment.

Supplementary microbiological diagnosis is useful in aggressive forms of periodontitis, as the success of mechanical therapy is questionable by high proportions of A. actinomycetem-comitans, P. gingivalis and B. forsythus. There is an international consensus that these microbes are oral pathogens (cf. Zambon, 1996).

In addition to the elimination of supragingival plaque and calculus, all diseased subgingival root surfaces must be carefully cleaned so as to support the body's own therapeutic processes sufficiently for full healing to take place. The efficacy of the measure described as root surface cleaning (deep scaling, root planing) has been documented by a large number of authors in randomized comparative clinical trials (RCTs) (see Table 8-2).

Table 8-2: Selection of comparative clinical trials[1] on the efficacy of subgingival root surface cleaning (deep scaling)				
Author	Year	Type	Duration (months)	Patients (n)
Hill	1981	RCT	24	90
Pihlstrom	1981	RCT	6/48	17
Nordland	1987	Cohorts	24	19
Becker	1988	RCT	12	16
Kaldahl	1988	RCT	3	82
Loos	1989	Cohorts	24	12

[1] A total of some 30 relevant studies on this subject (source: Ann Periodontol 1 [1996], pp. 443–490)

These studies showed that careful subgingival cleaning was enough to obtain a treatment result of similar quality to that possible in combination with surgical methods (cf. Pihlstrom, Ortiz & McHugh, 1981). It is well known that even where very deep pockets are initially present, a residual probing depth of 4 mm can be achieved by this method (cf. Knowles et al., 1979; Badersten, Nilvéus & Egelberg, 1981; 1984a; 1984b; 1985a; 1985b; 1985c; 1985d; 1987).

This stage of treatment is followed by a re-evaluation in which all teeth are subjected to a further thorough clinical examination for bleeding residual pockets.

8.3 Additional (surgical) treatment

If examination reveals the presence of residual infected pockets or furcation involvement, further periodontal treatment must be planned. Surgical methods are used to eliminate the residual bacterial deposits and granulation tissue, and corrective measures are applied either to initiate regeneration of the lost attachment apparatus or for further improvement of the dentition's own hygiene capacity.

A number of different methods of periodontal surgery are available for the additional treatment (see Table 8-3). The meta-analysis of Antczak-Bouckoms et al. (1993) shows that surgery can achieve a further reduction in probing depth in the case of deep residual pockets, whereas additional attachment loss is likely to occur at sites with shallow pockets (cf. Antczak-Bouckoms, 1993; Antczak-Bouckoms et al., 1993).

Table 8-3: Periodontal surgical procedures for the treatment of defects due to inflammation	
1. Resective procedures for pocket elimination or reduction	Apical sliding flap or apically repositioned flap with/without – bone resection – distal wedge excision gingivectomy (external or internal) access flaps (modified Widman flaps)
2. Regenerative procedures	Regenerative therapy (GTR) using: – transplants – implants (membranes) – growth proteins
3. Furcation therapy	tunnelling hemisection, radectomy

A number of comparative studies prove the advantages of regenerative treatment (GTR), although the prospects of success vary with the morphology of the defect and/or with the affected tooth (cf. Laurell & Gottlow, 1998). For instance, Proestakis et al. (1992) observed no definite difference between regeneratively treated sites and teeth that had received conventional therapy. Regenerative treatment was shown to have clear advantages in the therapy of degree II mandibular furcation defects and degree II furcation defects of the buccal surfaces of the upper molars (cf. Pontoriero & Lindhe, 1995; Pontoriero et al., 1987; Pontoriero et al.,1988; 1989).

Regular maintenance care after completion of corrective treatment is of crucial importance for the long-term success of the therapy as a whole. It has been known for over 20 years that regular recall (at intervals of three to six months) can prevent further tooth loss over a period of two decades (!) – in other words, depending on the regularity of maintenance care and the extent of the patient's cooperation, over 90% of affected teeth can be retained (cf. Axelsson & Lindhe, 1981a; 1981b; Axelsson, Lindhe & Nyström, 1991; Hirschfeld & Wasserman, 1978; McFall, 1982). The comparative study by Axelsson & Lindhe (1981a) showed that a rapid relapse accompanied by further attachment loss occurs in the absence of maintenance care.

8.4 Conclusion

Recent large-scale studies in the United States have demonstrated that periodontitis may influence the general health status and that, for example, the risk of premature birth or the birth of an underweight baby is increased by a factor of up to 6 in pregnant women with severe generalized periodontitis. It is now likewise accepted that periodontitis aggravates the risk of cardiac infarction and cardiovascular diseases (such as strokes) (cf. Beck et al., 1996; Beck et al., 1998; Offenbacher et al., 1996; Offenbacher et al., 1998; Page et al., 1997; Salvi et al., 1997).

In so far as scientific evidence ought to be the foundation of our practical activity, the implications for periodontology in the German legal health insurance scheme are a need for radical rethinking and the introduction of a long overdue reform – which, notwithstanding many years of pleading by the scientific society competent for our specialty, has been obstructed by the responsible politicians again and again.

These measures alone will not suffice, as a shift of emphasis in practical dental activity will be necessary at the same time. The current dominance of restorative measures should be relinquished in favour of early diagnosis, prevention and conservation.

Dentists today are still not trained with these considerations in mind. Restorative measures continue to predominate in dental studies, which are substantially based on the perspectives of the 1970s (!). Preventive aspects, such as periodontology, account for only an insignificant and not clearly defined proportion of the overall curriculum. Precisely the subgingival cleaning of infected root surfaces (deep scaling), whose efficacy cannot be overestimated, calls for intensive training owing to the demanding technique involved. A reform of dental education would contribute in the medium term to a clear shift of emphasis in dental practice and make for an even better level of health among our population.

A detailed survey of scientific evidence in our specialty is beyond the scope of this paper. A number of excellent reviews in the field have appeared in the last few years. Those deserving of particular mention here include the summary of the last World Workshop on Clinical Periodontics and the reports on the European workshops published by Quintessenz. In addition, up-to-date literature reviews on specific topics are presented on an ongoing basis by the journal "Periodontology 2000".

8.5 Literatur/References

Antczak-Bouckoms, A.: Meta-analysis of clinical trials in periodontal research. Periodontol 2000 2 (1993), 140–149

Antczak-Bouckoms, A., Joshipura, K., Burdick, E., Tulloch, J. F. C.: Meta-analysis of surgical versus non-surgical methods of treatment for periodontal disease. J Clin Periodontol 20 (1993), 259–268

Axelsson, P., Lindhe, J.: The significance of maintenance care in the treatment of periodontal disease. J Clin Periodontol 8 (1981a), 281–294

Axelsson, P., Lindhe, J.: Effect of controlled oral hygiene procedures on caries and periodontal disease in adults. Results after 6 years. J Clin Periodontol 8 (1981b), 239–248

Axelsson, P., Lindhe, J., Nyström, B.: On the prevention of caries and periodontal disease. Results of a 15-year longitudinal study in adults. J Clin Periodontol 18 (1991), 182–189

Badersten, A., Nilvéus, R., Egelberg, J.: Effect of nonsurgical periodontal therapy. I. Moderately advanced periodontitis. J Clin Periodontol 8 (1981), 57–72

Badersten, A., Nilvéus, R., Egelberg, J.: Effect of nonsurgical periodontal therapy. II. Severely advanced periodontitis. J Clin Periodontol 11 (1984a), 63–76

Badersten, A., Nilvéus, R., Egelberg, J.: Effect of nonsurgical periodontal therapy. III. Single versus repeated instrumentation. J Clin Periodontol 11 (1984b), 114–124

Badersten, A., Nilvéus, R., Egelberg, J.: Effect of nonsurgical periodontal therapy. IV. Operator variability. J Clin Periodontol 12 (1985a), 190–200

Badersten, A., Nilvéus, R., Egelberg, J.: Effect of nonsurgical periodontal therapy. V. Patterns of probing attachment loss in non-responding sites. J Clin Periodontol 12 (1985b), 270–282

Badersten, A., Nilvéus, R., Egelberg, J.: Effect of nonsurgical periodontal therapy. VI. Localization of sites with probing attachment loss. J Clin Periodontol 12 (1985c), 351–359

Badersten, A., Nilvéus, R., Egelberg, J.: Effect of nonsurgical periodontal therapy. VII. Bleeding, suppuration and probing depth in sites with probing attachment loss. J Clin Periodontol 12 (1985d), 432–440

Badersten, A., Nilvéus, R., Egelberg, J.: Effect of nonsurgical periodontal therapy. VIII. Probing attachment changes related to clinical characteristics. J Clin Periodontol 14 (1987), 425–432

Beck, J., Garcia, R., Heiss, G., Vokonas, P. S., Offenbacher, S.: Periodontal disease and cardiovascular disease. J Periodontol 67 (1996), 1123

Beck, J. D., Offenbacher, S., Williams, R., Gibbs, P., Garcia, R.: Periodontitis: a risk factor for coronary heart disease? Ann Periodontol 3 (1998), 127

Haffajee, A. D., Socransky, S. S.: Attachment level changes in destructive periodontal diseases. J Clin Periodontol 13 (1986), 461

Hirschfeld, L., Wasserman, B.: A long-term survey of tooth loss in 600 treated periodontal patients. J Periodontol 49 (1978), 225–237

Knowles, J. W., Burgett, F. G., Nissle, R. R., Shick, R. A., Morrison, E. C., Ramfjord, S. P.: Results of periodontal treatment related to pocket depth and attachment level. Eight years. J Periodontol 50 (1979), 225

8.5 Literatur/References

Laurell, L., Gottlow, J.: Guided tissue regeneration update. Int Dent J 48 (1998), 386

McFall, W. T.: Tooth loss in 100 treated patients with periodontal disease. A long-term study. J Periodontol 53 (1982), 539

Nyman, S., Lindhe, J., Rosling, B.: Periodontal surgery in plaque-infected dentitions. J Clin Periodontol 4 (1977), 240

Offenbacher, S., Jared, H. L., O'Reilly, P. G., Wells, S. R., Salvi, G. E., Lawrence, H. P., Socransky, S. S., Beck, J. D.: Potential pathogenic mechanisms of periodontitis associated pregnancy complications. Ann Periodontol 3 (1998), 233

Offenbacher, S., Katz, V., Fertik, G., Collins, J., Boyd, D., Maynor, G., McKaig, R., Beck, J.: Periodontal infection as a possible risk factor for preterm low birth weight. J Periodontol 67 (1996), 1103

Page, R. C., Offenbacher, S., Schroeder, H. E., Seymour, G. J., Kornman, K. S.: Advances in the pathogenesis of periodontitis: summary of developments, clinical implications and future directions. Periodontol 2000 14 (1997), 216

Pihlstrom, B. L., Ortiz, C. C., McHugh, R. B.: A randomized four-years study of periodontal therapy. J Periodontol 52 (1981), 227

Pontoriero, R., Lindhe, J.: Guided tissue regeneration in the treatment of degree III furcation defects in maxillary molars. J Clin Periodontol 22 (1995), 810

Pontoriero, R., Lindhe, J., Nyman, S., Karring, T., Rosenberg, E., Sanavi, F.: Guided tissue regeneration in degree II furcation-involved mandibular molars. A clinical study. J Clin Periodontol 15 (1988), 247

Pontoriero, R., Lindhe, J., Nyman, S., Karring, T., Rosenberg, E., Sanavi, F.: Guided tissue regeneration in the treatment of furcation defects in mandibular molars. A clinical study of degree III involvements. J Clin Periodontol 16 (1989), 170

Pontoriero, R., Nyman, S., Lindhe, J., Rosenberg, E., Sanavi, F.: Guided tissue regeneration in the treatment of furcation defects in man. J Clin Periodontol 14 (1987), 618

Proestakis, G., Bratthall, G., Soderholm, G., Kullendorff, B., Grondahl, K., Rohlin, M., Attstrom, R.: Guided tissue regeneration in the treatment of infrabony defects on maxillary premolars. A pilot study. J Clin Periodontol 19 (1992), 766–773

Richards, D., Lawrence, A., Sackett, D. L.: Bringing an evidence-base to dentistry [Editorial]. Community Dent Health 14 (1997), 63

Sackett, D. L.: Evidence-based medicine [Editorial]. Spine 23 (1998), 1085

Salvi, G. E., Yalda, B., Collins, J. G., Jones, B. H., Smith, F. W., Arnold, R. R., Offenbacher, S.: Inflammatory mediator response as a potential risk marker for periodontal diseases in insulin-dependent diabetes mellitus patients. J Periodontol 68 (1997), 127

Zambon, J. J.: Periodontal diseases: microbial factors. Ann Periodontol 1 (1996), 879

9 Brauchen wir neue Forschungsstrategien in der Zahn-, Mund- und Kieferheilkunde?

Wilfried Wagner, Mainz

9.1 Einleitung

Begriffe wie z. B. „prospektiv randomisierte Therapievergleichsstudien", „Meta-Analysen" und deren Auswertung erfahren nicht zuletzt durch die Diskussion um die Evidenz wissenschaftlicher Aussagen in der Medizin und die politischen Veränderungen im Gesundheitswesen allgemeine Beachtung. „Evidence-Based Medicine" (EBM) ist dabei der allgemein gebräuchliche, umfassende, richtige Ausdruck, wobei in diesem Begriff auch die Zahnmedizin betrachtet werden muss (vgl. Kerschbaum, 2000; Meyle, 2000; Reich, 2000; Reinert und Krimmel, 2000). Auch wenn im Rahmen dieser Publikation, in einem Teil der Literatur und zum Teil sogar als offizielle Bezeichnung für entsprechende Institute „Evidence-Based Dentistry" eingeführt wird, ist dies nur als Teilbegriff der evidenz-basierten Medizin zu betrachten, da Zahnmedizin immer ein Teil der Medizin ist. Auch für die anderen Fachgebiete der Medizin werden keine eigenständigen Bezeichnungen, sondern maximal Unterbegriffe eingeführt. Durch EBM werden hohe Erwartungen geweckt: In der Frankfurter Allgemeinen Zeitung vom 31.12.1997 findet man die Überschrift eine „Reformbewegung für die Kranken" oder gar „ein neues Zeitalter der Medizin". Dabei stellt sich selbstverständlich auch die Frage, ob dies Auswirkungen auf künftige Forschungsstrategien in der Zahnheilkunde haben wird.

9.2 Definition und methodische Begrenzung

Mit dem insbesondere von David L. Sackett eingeführten bzw. propagierten Begriff der Evidence-Based Medicine (EBM) wird seit ca. den 70er-Jahren zunehmend die wissenschaftliche Absicherung von Entscheidungsabläufen in der Medizin auf der Basis klinisch-wissenschaftlicher Studien beschrieben und methodisch aufgearbeitet. Sackett selbst definiert sie als „den gewissenhaften, ausdrücklichen und vernünftigen Gebrauch der gegenwärtig besten externen wissenschaftlichen Evidenz" für Entscheidungen in der medizinischen Versorgung individueller Patienten (vgl. Sackett et al., 1997). Im Gegensatz dazu wird die individuelle professionelle Erfahrung als erfahrene Sachkompetenz bzw. als „innere Evidenz" bezeichnet.

Die Methodik der EBM beschäftigt sich vor allem mit klinischen Fragestellungen und klinischen Studien und graduiert die wissenschaftliche Absicherung in unterschiedliche Evidenzgrade in Abhängigkeit von der Qualität der zu Grunde liegenden Studien (vgl. Tab. 9-1). Evidenz-basierte Medizin ist eine Qualitätssicherungsstrategie für medizinische Entscheidungsabläufe, die entwickelt wurde und die weiterentwickelt wird als wissenschaftlich-systematische Methodik, um klinisch-wissenschaftliche Forschung für Entscheidungsprozesse als bestmögliche externe Evidenz nutzbar zu machen (vgl. Porzolt und Kunz, 1997). Mit diesen Maßnahmen lässt sich nur ein kleiner, aber wichtiger Teilbereich der Forschung absichern, der sich mit klinischen Studien beschäftigt. Da aber die klinische Forschung im Mittelpunkt der Evidenzgraduierung steht, sind entsprechend der Graduierung sekundär Rückwirkungen auf die Forschungsstrategien – gerade auf die klinische Forschung – zu erwarten. Reich schreibt, dass bezüglich der klinischen Validität der Aussagen von Studien neue methodische Strategien entwickelt werden müssen, welche die Aussagekraft von klinischen Studien verbessern (vgl. Reich, 2000). Die systematische Aufarbeitung und Bewertung der klinischen Forschung in einer methodisch reproduzierbaren Weise ist der wesentliche und wichtige Beitrag der EBM für die Medizin und damit auch für die Zahnmedizin.

Es gibt aber einen wichtigen Teil an Forschung, der als Grundlagenforschung darüber hinausgeht, der nicht mit EBM-Kriterien zu fassen ist und nicht in die vorgegebenen klinisch orientierten Evidenzgrade hineinpasst.

Tabelle 9-1: Einteilung der Evidenzstärke nach AHCPR (Agency for Health Care Policy and Research), 1992	
Grad	Evidenz-Typ
Ia	Evidenz aufgrund von Meta-Analysen randomisierter, kontrollierter Studien
Ib	Evidenz aufgrund mindestens einer randomisierten, kontrollierten Studie
IIa	Evidenz aufgrund mindestens einer gut angelegten, kontrollierten Studie ohne Randomisierung
IIb	Evidenz aufgrund mindestens einer gut angelegten, quasi-experimentellen Studie
III	Evidenz aufgrund gut angelegter, nicht experimenteller deskriptiver Studien (z. B. Vergleichsstudien, Korrelationsstudien, Fall-Kontrollstudien)
IV	Evidenz aufgrund von Berichten/Meinungen von Expertenkreisen, Konsensuskonferenzen und/oder klinischer Erfahrung anerkannter Autoritäten
Quelle: ÄZQ, 1999	

Auch die kritischen Stimmen von v. Uexküll und Herrmann, die der in der EBM erfassten „pragmatischen Evidenz" die in ihren Augen umfassendere „kommunikative Evidenz" entgegenstellen, müssen bei aller Euphorie bedacht werden (siehe hierzu auch Kapitel 4).

Im Deutschen Ärzteblatt vom November 1999 wird ferner ein ganz anderes Problem der EBM-Diskussion deutlich gemacht, der Einfluss kultureller Faktoren auf die entsprechenden medizinischen Entscheidungen – und natürlich auch auf entsprechende Studien – am Beispiel der Einstellung zur prophylaktischen Mammaresektion in Frankreich und in den Vereinigten Staaten (vgl. Meyer, 1999). Weil in diesen Ländern das Organ mit unterschiedlicher kulturell-symbolischer und ästhetischer Bedeutung belegt ist, wurden sehr unterschiedliche, scheinbar evidenz-basierte, gesicherte Rückschlüsse aus den Daten gezogen. Neben der EBM gibt es also auch die Einflüsse einer „Culture-Based Medicine (CBM)".

9.3 Notwendigkeit von EBM-Kriterien in Abhängigkeit der Wirksamkeit

Der Begriff der „offensichtlichen Wirksamkeit" in Bezug zu den geforderten Evidenzgraden ist ein besonders wichtiges Thema. Die Frage der Wirksamkeit, der Offensichtlichkeit, muss natürlich auch Einfluss darauf haben, wie hoch die Anforderung an den Evidenzgrad ist. Methoden mit geringem Unterschied brauchen einen hohen Evidenzgrad, und bei offensichtlich wirksamen Methoden reicht ein ganz niedriger Evidenzgrad, unter Umständen sogar nur mit einigen Fallberichten. Ein gutes Beispiel ist die Methodik der Kallusdistraktion. Für die Kallusdistraktion gibt es gute experimentelle Studien, aber keinesfalls prospektiv randomisierte Studien, und trotzdem würde heute jeder eine entsprechende Hypoplasie im Unterkiefer bei einem Kleinkind statt mit Beckenkamm-Osteoplastik mit der Kallusdistraktion therapieren. Weil die Effektivität dieser Therapie so hoch und die Belastung geringer ist, kommt es zu einem breiten klinischen Einsatz, ohne dass man hier einen Evidenzgrad einer prospektiv randomisierten Studie fordern würde.

9.4 Gefahren von EBM-Kriterien

Selektion
EBM-Forschung hat selbst ihren methodischen Bias, da randomisierte Studien in der Regel strenge Einschluss- und Ausschlusskriterien haben, um die Homogenität der zu vergleichenden Gruppen zu sichern. Darin aber liegt eine wesentliche Selektion der Therapiegruppen. Und was wir dann in diesen randomisierten Selektionsstudien ermitteln, ist nicht ohne weiteres allgemein gültig, sondern ist nur allgemein gültig für diese definierten Patientengruppen. Man darf nicht erwarten, dass die dort beschriebenen

Tabelle 9-2: Forschungsstrategie (begrenzende Fachprobleme)
– Häufigkeit (z. B.: sehr seltene Krankheitsbilder)
– Therapiewandel (z. B.: Materialneuentwicklungen)
– Einwilligung (z. B.: Randomisierung Eltern)
– individuelle Variationsbreite (z. B.: Tumor)
– Langzeitbeobachtungen (z. B.: LKG-Therapie)
– subjektive Bewertungskriterien (z. B.: Ästhetik)
– Aktualität (z. B.: Distraktionsosteogenese)

98%igen Erfolgsraten z. B. in der Implantologie auf ein dann nicht mehr selektioniertes Krankengut übertragbar sind, und es werden möglicherweise damit falsche Rückschlüsse auf die Effektivität einer Maßnahme abgeleitet.

Methodische Begrenzungen und Wissenschaftsmanipulation
Es bestehen auch methodische Begrenzungen (vgl. Tab. 9-2) durch Beschränkung bestimmter Fragestellungen auf einzelne Fachthemen. Darüber hinaus entsteht die Gefahr der Wissenschaftsmanipulation durch eine industriell genutzte, nur scheinbar objektive Wissenschaft, die durch gezielte Aufträge mit entsprechenden Studien als Marketing für ein bestimmtes Produkt die sogenannte klinische Absicherung erkauft und missbraucht.

9.5 Rückwirkung der EBM auf die Forschung

Evidenz-basierte Medizin wird durch die Konzentrierung auf klinische Studien und Meta-Analysen auch Rückwirkungen auf die künftige Forschungsstrategie haben (vgl. Perleth, 1998). Es wird nur eine Frage der Zeit sein, bis

Tabelle 9-3: Traditionelle und künftige Forschungsstrategie	
traditionell	künftig
– klinische Prüfung	– prospektive Therapievergleich-Studien
– neue Werkstoffe	– Randomisierung
– Implantatsysteme	– Multicenter-Studien
– Technologie	– Forschungsverbund mit zahnärztlichen Praxen
– Grundlagenforschung	– professionelle Meta-Analysen
– Werkstoffprüfung	(systematische Übersichtsarbeiten)
– Zellkultur	– wissenschaftliche Literaturaufbereitung als
– Tierexperiment	Dienstleistung
– Molekularbiologie	

Geldflüsse für Forschungsförderung an EBM-Kriterien angekoppelt werden, und dann wird die traditionelle Forschung auch in diese Richtung künftig klinisch orientierter Forschung (vgl. Tab. 9-3) gelenkt. Das kann sinnvoll sein für viele Bereiche, in denen eine solche systematische klinische Forschung notwendig und möglich ist, aber die Forschung darf sich nicht ausschließlich darauf konzentrieren.

Im letzten Jahr wurde z. B. von der DGZMK mit 250.000 DM zellorientierte, molekularbiologische Grundlagenforschung gefördert, was ein ebenso wichtiger Teilbereich in der Forschung für unser Fach ist. Bei aller Begeisterung für die EBM, die auch durch eine sicher übertriebene Erwartungshaltung in der Politik und bei den Kostenträgern in Bezug auf mögliche Einspareffekte durch die Konzentration auf Evidenzkriterien verstärkt wurde, darf die Grundlagenforschung im Experiment und Labor nicht zurückgenommen werden.

Gute klinische Forschung und prospektiv randomisierte Studien (vgl. Egger, Zellweger und Antes, 1996) sind meist zeit- und kostenaufwendig, so dass auch die finanziellen Fragen der klinischen Studien angesprochen werden müssen. Die Einrichtung der Zentren für klinische Forschung an den Hochschulen ist ein erster Schritt in diese Richtung. Gerade junge Nachwuchswissenschaftler müssen für die eher auf Langzeitbeobachtung angelegten Studien ohne kurzfristig publizierbare Ergebnisse gewonnen werden, wozu in der Zahnmedizin aufgrund des engen akademischen Mittelbaus die Voraussetzungen eher ungünstig sind.

9.6 Veränderungen in der zahnmedizinischen Forschung durch EBM-Strategien

Es bestehen Gefahren in der evidenz-basierten Medizin, wenn man nicht das Gesamtbild der Forschung betrachtet, und zum Gesamtbild der Forschung gehört ganz wesentlich die traditionelle Grundlagenforschung. In der zahnärztlichen Werkstoffkunde gibt es viel – allerdings eher mechanistisch orientierte – Literatur, wobei die Materialien inzwischen auch Zellkul-

Tabelle 9-4: Studiendesignbildungen
– In-vitro-Studien
– tierexperimentelle Studien
– Fallberichte
– retrospektive Querschnittsstudien
– prospektive Longitudinalstudien
– prospektiv randomisierte Therapievergleichsstudien
– prospektiv randomisierte Doppelblindstudien

turprüfungen unterzogen werden. Wenn aber unter Grundlagenforschung auch molekularbiologische und molekulare Basisaspekte gesehen werden, dann wird die Literaturbasis in der Zahnheilkunde bereits dünn, und es besteht dort ein mindestens ebenso hoher Forschungsbedarf wie bei randomisierten klinischen Verlaufsstudien.

EBM-Strategien werden die klinische Forschung bzw. methodische Designfragen verändern (vgl. Tab. 9-4). Die klinischen Prüfungen, die in der Vergangenheit viel zu häufig reine Anwendungsbeobachtungen waren – und keine ausreichend randomisierten prospektiven Studien –, werden sich nicht zuletzt durch die Diskussion um EBM im positiven Sinne ändern. Nun kann man sagen, dass die Schwierigkeit, solche Studien durchzuführen, zunimmt, und zwar vom niedrigen bis zum hohem Evidenzgrad, so dass im Allgemeinen auch der deduktive Wert oder die Verallgemeinerungsberechtigung zunimmt. Am Beispiel der Doppelblindstudie lässt sich aber aufzeigen, dass häufig einfach methodische Grenzen bestehen. Grenzen bestehen auch, die in den Ausführungen zur kommunikativen Evidenz (siehe hierzu auch Kapitel 4) sehr deutlich angesprochen wurden: Die Entscheidung, ob die Therapie A oder B durchgeführt wird, hängt zu einem ganz wesentlichen Teil auch von den Patienten ab.

Es erhebt sich weiterhin die Frage des Kostenrahmens für randomisierte Studien, wenn man z. B. unterschiedliche Kosten für zwei Therapieverfahren mit einem Faktor 5-10 hat, wie dies am Beispiel der Implantologie möglich ist. Es liegen nicht einmal gute, wirklich randomisierte Studien vor, die nach EBM-Kriterien den Unterschied zwischen einer polierten und nicht polierten Amalgamfüllung belegen. Dies ist eine von vielen ganz einfachen Fragen, deren Beantwortung viel Mühe und Kosten bereiten würde. Eine randomisierte vergleichende Studie mit vielen Tausend Amalgamfüllungen kann beeindrucken, liefert aber keinen Beleg über die Qualität dieser Amalgamfüllungen. Am anderen Beispiel einer aufwendigen, adhäsiven Füllungstechnik mit Klammern, mit Kofferdam, mit Keilen und vielen Dingen mehr wird das Problem der Detailfragen besonders deutlich. Welche dieser Maßnahmen, die quasi als Dogmen übernommen wurden und sich als state of the art zur Durchführung einer solchen Therapie in den Lehrbüchern finden, ist mit einem Evidenzgrad belegt? Es ist ein Fehler zu glauben, alle Fragen der Zahnmedizin seien mit dem Zauberwort EBM zu lösen. Zur sinnvollen

Tabelle 9-5: Priorisierungsliste

- allgemeine Bedeutung des Problems
- Häufigkeit des Problems
- Divergenz der Meinungen
- mangelnde Absicherung
- Zugänglichkeit oder Möglichkeit der Absicherung

Forschungsplanung sind bei begrenzten Ressourcen Priorisierungsstrategien erforderlich, welche Fragen wir mit welchem Evidenzgrad in klinischen Untersuchungen lösen können oder lösen sollen (vgl. Tab. 9-5).

Dabei muss ein Punkt deutlich angesprochen werden: Wenn EBM aus randomisierten Studien akzeptiert werden soll, dann müssen die Fragen eines Forschungsnetzwerks zwischen Praxis und Klinik gelöst werden. Übertragbare Ergebnisse können nicht gewonnen werden, wenn nur in einer randomisierten kleinen Gruppe unter hochspeziellen Bedingungen die Therapie durchgeführt wird. Nur mit einer wirklich großen Fallzahl und mit unterschiedlichen strukturellen Ausgangsbedingungen wird die notwendige Akzeptanz der Ergebnisse auch in der alltäglichen Praxissituation erreicht. Man erfährt auch vor allen Dingen, inwieweit die Routine Einfluss auf zwei miteinander zu vergleichende Methoden hat. Aber es besteht dabei das Problem des Aufwands, der Datenerfassung und des unmittelbaren Nutzens für die unterschiedlichen Behandler und vor allem für die Patienten. Es müssen neue Forschungsstrategien entstehen, und es gilt zu überlegen, wie diese Partnerschaft Praxis-Klinik und Patient-Behandler für solche Studien in einer sinnvollen Weise aktiviert werden kann.

9.7 Detailprobleme randomisierter Studien in der Zahnheilkunde

Prospektive randomisierte Studien werden durch die technischen Entwicklungen gerade in der Zahnheilkunde durch neue Materialien und Methoden in ihrer Bedeutung reduziert. So ist eine der prospektiv randomisierten Multicenter-Studien trotz DFG-Förderung über viele Jahre aus formalistischen Gründen noch nicht veröffentlicht, weil die Methodiker sie immer noch auf ihre statistische Aussagefähigkeit überprüfen. Aber alle drei Teilstudien beschreiben Implantate, die inzwischen durch Neuentwicklungen abgelöst wurden und nicht mehr im Markt verfügbar sind.

Ein weiteres Problem stellt das Zielkriterium solcher Studien dar. So war z. B. für die Implantate im zahnlosen Unterkiefer das Überleben der Implantate das Hauptzielkriterium, und hier zeigte sich kein Unterschied. Aber was ist das Zielkriterium der randomisierten Studie? Das Zielkriterium ist auch bei der onkologischen Forschung längst nicht mehr nur das Überleben, sondern auch die Frage der psychosozialen Lebensqualität in dieser Zeit des Überlebens und danach, ob es andere Vorteile gibt. Insofern müssen bei randomisierten Studien nicht einfache Analysen, sondern die Begleitfaktoren und Befunde differenzierter betrachtet werden, und dann werden die Dinge viel schwieriger. In der obigen Studie wurde nicht nur die Frage Implantate in situ, sondern zusätzliche Faktoren, wie Knochenabbau und Taschen analysiert, und nun ist plötzlich doch ein Unterschied zwischen den Gruppen entstanden, der in einer Gruppe einen deutlicheren Abfall des Anteils der völlig reizlosen Implantate gegenüber der anderen Gruppe zeigt.

Oder eine andere Detailfrage: Eine Studie mit vier ITI-Implantaten, alle 12 mm lang und alle mit einem gleichen Durchmesser erhielten randomisiert einen normalem Steg und die andere Gruppe einen Extensionssteg. Auch hier zeigten sich keine Unterschiede im Überleben, aber eine bei Beginn der Studie noch unbekannte Variable der Knochenhöhe hinter den Implantaten zeigte signifikante Unterschiede, die bei einer Entwicklung zur Neugestaltung der präventionsorientierten Zahnheilkunde wesentlich im Therapievergleich sind. Das Zielkriterium solcher Studien muss ggf. adaptiert werden.

Es bleiben viele Fragen offen, wie auch die der angemessenen Versorgung für die Lösung des gleichen Problems, nämlich einer implantatprothetischen Versorgung des zahnlosen Unterkiefers. Vergleicht man unterschiedliche implantatprothetische Versorgungen miteinander, so kommt bei der Auswahl der geeigneten Versorgungsform auch wieder die kommunikative Evidenz, aber auch die intrinsische Evidenz des Behandlers hinzu.

Die Frage der Häufigkeit stellt in der Zahnheilkunde meist kein Problem dar, da Karies- und Parodontalerkrankungen oder Implantate in einer ausreichenden Häufigkeit auftreten. Aber es müssen auch seltene Krankheitsbilder durch ggf. internationale Multicenter-Strategien einbezogen werden.

Das Problem der Randomisierung besteht jedoch insbesondere, wenn Kinder betroffen sind. Eltern willigen nur sehr selten zur Randomisierung ein, weil sie natürlich die jeweils bessere Therapie für ihr Kind wollen. Die individuelle Variationsbreite wird am Beispiel des Tumors sehr deutlich.

Besonders hinderlich sind Probleme der Langzeitbeobachtung, insbesondere bei Therapien, die das Wachstum beeinflussen, wie am Beispiel der Therapie von Lippen-Kiefer-Gaumenspalten bei Patienten von über 18 Jahren deutlich wird. Die Frage des subjektiven Therapienutzens wird am Beispiel der Ästhetik besonders deutlich, und es bleibt die Frage der Aktualität oder der offensichtlichen Wirksamkeit. Es gibt eine große europäische Multicenter-Studie, die die Therapie von Lippen-Kiefer-Gaumenspalten vergleicht, wobei vor allem analysiert wurde, welche Auswirkungen auf das skelettale Wachstum entstanden sind. Als einzige stringente Variable kam heraus, dass die Erfahrung des Behandlers, d.h. die intrinsische Evidenz, viel wichtiger war als die Methodik. Daraus zieht man im englischen Gesundheitssystem den Schluss, dass man die Behandlungszentren auf wenige, mit jeweils über 20 Kindern pro Jahr, begrenzt.

Man wird die Strategien im Hinblick auf dafür zugängliche Fragen sicher in Zukunft adaptieren müssen, um damit die Qualität der Aussagen, auf die wir uns stützen, zu verbessern. Im letzten Supplement Evidence-based Dentistry des British Dental Journal (1999) werden zwei von der Cochrane Oral Health Group abgeschlossene Reviews veröffentlicht: „Orthodontic treatments for posterior crossbites" (Harrison, J., Asby, D.) und zur Therapie des

Lichen ruber „Interventions for treating oral lichen planus" (Chan, E., Thornhill, M., Zakrzewska, J.).

Der letztgenannte Review enthält eine Literaturauswertung zu den Therapieformen der Intervention beim Lichen ruber planus. Es wurden dort insgesamt 9 Studien zu 4 Gruppen (Cyclosporin, Retinoide, Steroide und Fototherapie) verglichen. Man hat sich auf diese hochwertigen, prospektiv randomisierten Studien beschränkt. Es wurde eine schwache Evidenz für die Wirksamkeit aller Methoden, aber kein Unterschied gefunden. Man kam zu dem Schluss, dass weitere standardisierte, sorgfältig selektierte Studien benötigt werden. Wenn man zusätzlich die nicht randomisierten Studien gründlich analysiert hätte, hätte man vielleicht auch die wichtige Frage der Unterschiede noch geklärt.

9.8 Bedeutung der EBM für die zahnärztliche Qualitätssicherung

Ganz ohne Frage sind die EBM-Methoden ein wichtiger Beitrag auch zur Qualitätssicherung der zahnärztlichen Arbeit, in dem Sinne, dass Fachleute sich die Mühe machen, Literatur zu sondieren, zu werten und aufzuarbeiten, damit sie den Kollegen in der Praxis sowie auch für entsprechende Verlautbarungen und für die Fortbildung als Basis dienen können. Neue akademische Berufsfelder sind zu erwarten, da die Informationsfülle der wissenschaftlichen Publikationen ohne professionelle Hilfe nicht zu bewerten und für die tägliche Arbeit zu integrieren ist. Hier ist die Cochrane Collaboration (vgl. Antes und Linde, 1995) als international agierende Bewegung sicher eine wichtige Einrichtung auf dem Feld der Qualitätssicherung. Diesen Gruppierungen wächst eine hohe Verantwortung – die Erstellung entsprechender wissenschaftlicher systematischer Reviews – zu; gleichermaßen muss ein solches neues wissenschaftliches Arbeitsfeld aber auch akademisch akzeptiert werden.

Betrachtet man die Literatur zu EBM (eine einfache Medline-Recherche, vgl. Tab. 9-6) dann sieht man den ansteigenden Anteil von Literaturstellen zu evidenz-basierter Medizin. Betrachtet man die Titel der evidenz-basier-

Tabelle 9-6: Ergebnis von Medline-Recherchen zu EBM und EBD		
Jahr	Evidence-Based Medicine	Evidence-Based Dentistry
	Anzahl Publikationen	
1996	214	5
1997	604	5
1998	951	7
1999	866	8

ten Zahnheilkunde, dann findet man insgesamt nur 25 Literaturstellen. Mit einer zeitlichen Verzögerung wird die Thematik auch in der zahnärztlichen Literatur aufgenommen.

9.9 Ausblick

Es werden gute, auf EBM-Kriterien gestützte Untersuchungen entwickelt. Sie werden auch die Forschungsstrategien in der klinischen Forschung zunehmend beeinflussen, weil sie zur Validierung der daraus gezogenen Schlussfolgerungen beitragen können. Insbesondere die klinische Forschung und der Umgang mit den internationalen Forschungsergebnissen wird sich entscheidend ändern. Aber dies ist nicht als eine isolierte Maßnahme zu sehen. Es bedarf eines multimodalen, kritischen Forschungsansatzes, wenn abgesicherte Entscheidungshilfen für Arzt und Patient für eine *zur Zeit wissenschaftlich abgesicherte*, angemessene Versorgung benötigt werden. Doch Arztsein ist mehr, als einen Patienten nur nach den letzten Erkenntnissen der evidenz-basierten Medizin zu behandeln, und Medizin ist mehr als die Summe von Naturwissenschaft und Technik (vgl. Diehl, 1999).

9 Do we need new research strategies in dentistry and oral medicine?

Wilfried Wagner, Mainz

9.1 Introduction

Partly owing to the debate about the evidence for scientific statements in medicine and the political changes in the health care system, general attention has been drawn to concepts such as "prospective randomized comparative therapeutic studies", "meta-analyses", and the evaluation of these investigations. "Evidence-based medicine" (EBM) is now accepted as the correct generic term for such an approach, and must be deemed to include dentistry (cf. Kerschbaum, 2000; Meyle, 2000; Reich, 2000; Reinert & Krimmel, 2000). Even if the term "evidence-based dentistry" has been introduced in the present publication, in some of the relevant literature and indeed, in some cases, in the official names of institutions working in this field, EBD must be regarded only as a sub-domain of evidence-based medicine, because dentistry is always a part of medicine. Specific denominations have not been introduced in other medical specialties, but only, at most, subsidiary concepts. EBM has aroused great expectations; for instance, headlines in the respected German newspaper Frankfurter Allgemeine Zeitung (31 Dec. 1997) proclaimed "A reform movement for patients" and even "A new era of medicine". The question of the possible repercussions on future research strategies in dentistry inevitably also arises.

9.2 Definition and methodological differentiation

The term "evidence-based medicine" (EBM) was introduced and propagated in particular by David L. Sackett and has been used increasingly since the 1970s to denote the scientific underpinning of decision-making processes in medicine on the basis of clinical-scientific studies and incorporation of the results in methodologies. Sackett himself defines EBM as "the conscientious, explicit and judicious use of current best external evidence" in making decisions about the medical care of individual patients (cf. Sackett et al., 1997). Conversely, individual professional experience is deemed to be the competence acquired by a practitioner in his field, or "internal evidence".

The methodology of EBM is concerned principally with clinical problems and studies and specifies the degree of scientific validation by different levels of evidence according to the quality of the studies on which it is based (cf. Table 9-1). Evidence-based medicine is a quality assurance strategy for medical decision-making processes that was developed, and is being further developed, as a systematic scientific methodology to allow clinical scientific research to be turned to account as the best possible external evidence for decision-making processes (cf. Porzolt & Kunz, 1997). Such measures can be used to underpin only a small – but important – area of research, namely that concerned with clinical studies. However, since clinical research is a focal point in the grading of evidence, the assigned level is likely to have secondary feedback effects on research strategies, and specifically on clinical research. According to Reich, new methodological strategies must be developed to improve the clinical validity of the results of clinical studies (cf. Reich, 2000). The systematic working-up and assessment of clinical research in a methodologically reproducible manner is EBM's essential and important contribution to medicine and hence also to dentistry.

However, beyond this field lies the important sphere of fundamental research, which does not lend itself to the application of EBM criteria and does not fit into the predetermined clinically oriented evidence validity classification. For all the euphoria, it is essential to bear in mind the criticisms voiced by von Uexküll and Herrmann, who contrast the "pragmatic evidence" that is the province of EBM with what they regard as the more comprehensive "communicative evidence" (see Chapter 4).

Table 9-1: Grading of evidence by the AHCPR (Agency for Health Care Policy and Research), 1992	
Level	Type of evidence
Ia	Evidence based on meta-analyses of randomized controlled studies
Ib	Evidence based on at least one randomized controlled study
IIa	Evidence based on at least one well designed controlled study without randomization
IIb	Evidence based on at least one well designed quasi-experimental study
III	Evidence based on well designed, non-experimental descriptive studies (e.g. comparative studies, correlation studies or case control studies)
IV	Evidence based on reports or opinions of expert groups, consensus conferences and/or clinical experience of recognized authorities
Source: ÄZQ, 1999	

The "Deutsches Ärzteblatt" for November 1999 highlights a completely different aspect of the EBM debate, namely the effect of cultural factors on medical decision-making and, of course, on the relevant studies. The example given relates to the differing attitudes to prophylactic breast resection prevailing in France and the United States (cf. Meyer, 1999). Since the cultural, symbolic and aesthetic significance of this organ differs as between the two countries, widely divergent seemingly evidence-based and validated conclusions are drawn from the data. Besides EBM, therefore, account must be taken of the influence of "culture-based medicine (CBM)".

9.3 Need for EBM criteria in relation to efficacy

The notion of "manifest efficacy" in relation to the levels of evidence demanded is a particularly important issue. The question of efficacy – of manifest effect – must of course also influence the degree of evidence demanded. Methods that differ only slightly need a high level of evidence, whereas a low degree – in some cases no more than a few case histories – suffices for manifestly effective methods. A good example is the callus distraction technique. Good experimental studies on callus distraction exist, but there are no prospective randomized studies – yet nowadays everyone would prefer this procedure to iliac crest osteoplasty for the treatment of mandibular hypoplasia in a very young child. Since this therapy is so effective and less invasive, its clinical use is widespread, and no one would demand the evidence level of a prospective randomized study for it.

9.4 Dangers of EBM criteria

Selection
EBM research has a methodological bias of its own, since randomized studies as a rule have strict inclusion and exclusion criteria in order to guarantee the homogeneity of the groups to be compared. However, this implies substantial selection of the therapy groups. The results of these studies do not then automatically possess general validity, but are valid generally only for these defined groups of patients. If such a study reports a 98% success rate in, e.g., implantology, there is no reason to expect such a figure to be applicable to an unselected group of patients, and it is quite possible for incorrect conclusions to be drawn about the efficacy of a measure.

Methodological limitations and the danger of manipulation of science
Further methodological limitations (see Table 9-2) arise when specific problems are considered only in terms of isolated issues. There is also the danger of scientific manipulation, where an industrial undertaking commissions research that is only seemingly objective and the relevant studies are used to market a given product; in this case the "clinical validation" has been purchased and misused.

Table 9-2: Research strategy (limitation to specific issues)
– Frequency (e.g. very rare clinical pictures)
– Changes in therapy (e.g. development of new materials)
– Consent (e.g. parental consent to randomization)
– Individual range of variation (e.g. tumours)
– Long-term observation (e.g. therapy of cheilognathopalatoschisis)
– Subjective evaluation criteria (e.g. aesthetics)
– Currency at a given time (e.g. distraction osteogenesis)

9.5 Feedback effects of EBM on research

Owing to its concentration on clinical studies and meta-analyses, evidence-based medicine will also have feedback effects on future research strategy (cf. Perleth, 1998). It is only a matter of time before research funding is made conditional on the application of EBM criteria, so that in the future traditional research will also tend to become clinically oriented (see Table 9-3). This may be appropriate for many fields, in which systematic clinical research of this kind is necessary and possible, but research must not be confined exclusively to this sphere.

Over the last year, for example, funds of some DM 250 000 were allocated by the DGZMK [German Society of Dentistry and Oral Medicine] to cell-oriented fundamental research in molecular biology, an equally important sub-domain of research in our discipline. For all the enthusiasm for EBM – no doubt reinforced by exaggerated expectations on the part of politicians and funding bodies of possible savings from the concentration on evidential

Table 9-3: Traditional and future research strategies	
Traditional	Future

– Clinical trials
  – new materials
  – implant systems
  – technology
	– Prospective comparative therapeutic studies
	– Randomization
	– Multi-centre studies
	– Joint research with dental practices

– Fundamental research
  – material testing
  – cell culture
  – animal experiments
  – molecular biology
	– Professional meta-analyses (systematic reviews)
	– Reviewing of scientific literature as a service

criteria – fundamental research at experimental and laboratory level must on no account be cut back.

Good clinical research and prospective randomized studies (cf. Egger, Zellweger & Antes, 1996) are usually time-consuming and expensive, so that the issue of the funding of clinical studies must also be addressed. The establishment of centres for clinical research at our universities is a first step in this direction. It is precisely the young generation of scientists who must be won over for studies based mainly on long-term observation, which do not yield short-term results for early publication; however, the lack of middle-level posts in the dental academic career structure militates against this.

9.6 Changes in dental research due to EBM strategies

Dangers lurk in evidence-based medicine unless the overall research picture is considered, and an essential aspect of this overall picture is traditional fundamental research. Most of the abundant literature on dental materials science is mechanically oriented, but some studies on cell-culture testing of materials do now exist. However, if fundamental research is deemed to include basic molecular and molecular-biology aspects, the literature base in the dental field is seen to be sparse, and the research requirement here proves to be at least as great as for randomized clinical long-term studies.

EBM strategies will modify clinical research and methodological design (see Table 9-4). Clinical trials, which in the past too often took the form purely of observations of applications rather than of adequately randomized prospective studies, will be modified in a positive sense partly by virtue of the EBM debate. The difficulty of conducting such studies may be said to increase from low to high levels of evidence, with, in general, a concomitant increase in deductive value or generalizability. However, the example of the double-blind study shows that simple methodological limitations sometimes obtain. Other limitations emerge clearly in the discussion of communicative evi-

Table 9-4: Types of study design
– In vitro studies
– Animal-experiment studies
– Case histories
– Retrospective cross-sectional studies
– Prospective longitudinal studies
– Prospective randomized comparative therapeutic studies
– Prospective randomized double-blind studies

Table 9-5: Priority list

- General importance of problem
- Frequency of problem
- Divergence of opinions
- Lack of validation
- Accessibility or possibility of validation

dence (see Chapter 4): not only the practitioner but also the patient makes an essential contribution to the decision to opt for therapy A or therapy B.

Another issue is the cost structure for randomized studies, where, for example, the cost of two therapeutic procedures differs by a factor of 5–10, as is possible in the case of implantology. We do not even have good, genuinely randomized studies based on EBM criteria that document the differences between polished and unpolished amalgam fillings. That is just one of a large number of very simple questions that could be answered only by the expenditure of a great deal of effort and money. A randomized comparative study covering thousands of amalgam fillings may be impressive but affords no proof of their quality. Problems of detail come into sharp focus in another example, that of expensive adhesive filling techniques using clamps, rubber dams, wedges and many other appurtenances. Which of these items, which are accepted virtually as dogma and have found their way into the textbooks as the state of the art for the conduct of such treatments, are supported by a level of evidence? It is a mistake to believe that all dental questions can be answered with the magic formula of EBM. Resources being limited, a sensible system of research planning calls for prioritization strategies to determine which problems can or should be solved on the basis of what level of evidence in clinical studies (see Table 9-5).

One point must be clearly addressed: if EBM based on randomized studies is to be accepted, the issue of a research network covering dental practices and clinics must be resolved. Transferable results cannot be obtained where therapy is undertaken only in a randomized small group under highly specific conditions. The necessary acceptance of the results, in everyday's dental practice situation, will be forthcoming only if the number of cases is really large and the initial structural conditions are diverse. Routine is found to be a major determinant of the choice between two alternative methods undergoing comparison. Other problems concern expenditure of time and effort, data acquisition, and the direct benefit to the various practitioners and, above all, to patients. New research strategies are necessary, and we must reflect on appropriate ways of activating this partnership between dental practice and clinic and between patient and practitioner for such studies.

9.7 Detailed problems of randomized studies in dentistry

Technical developments in dentistry in particular, due to new materials and methods, reduce the importance of prospective randomized studies. For instance, despite funding from the DFG [German Society for the Advancement of Scientific Research], one prospective randomized multi-centre study remains unpublished after many years for formalistic reasons, because the methodologists are still assessing its statistical validity. However, all three parts of the study describe implants since superseded by new products and no longer available on the market.

The target criterion of such studies is another problem. For example, the main target criterion in a study of implants in the edentulous mandible was survival of the implants, and here no difference was observed. But what is the target criterion of a randomized study? In oncology research, too, the target criterion has for a long time not been just survival as such, but also includes quality of life in the survival period and other possible benefits. In other words, randomized studies must not be mere analyses but should also take more differentiated account of attendant factors and findings – and then matters become much more difficult. The study mentioned above not only dealt with implants in situ but also analysed other factors, such as bone destruction and pockets, and then a difference between the groups did emerge: the proportion of completely irritation-free implants was found to be significantly less in one group than in the other.

Another question of detail concerns a study of four ITI implants, all 12 mm long and all with the same diameter. On a randomized basis, one group had ordinary abutments and the other extension abutments. Here again no differences in survival were found, but a variable as yet unknown when the study began, bone height behind the implants, did show significant variation. This is highly relevant when the therapies are compared for the purpose of revising preventive-dentistry recommendations. The target criterion of such studies must be adapted where necessary.

Many outstanding issues remain, e.g. the appropriate solution to the specific problem of prosthetic treatment of the edentulous mandible, comparing different implant solutions as a basis for prosthetic care. In deciding on the appropriate solution also the communicative evidence proves to be relevant – as well as the practitioner's intrinsic evidence.

Frequency is not usually a problem in dentistry, as carious and periodontal diseases or implants are frequent enough. However, rare clinical pictures must also be covered, where necessary by international multi-centre strategies.

The problem of randomization arises with particular force in the case of children. Parents seldom agree to randomization because they naturally want their child to have whatever therapy is best. The individual range of variation is revealed clearly by the example of tumours.

Problems of long-term observation are particularly awkward, especially in the case of growth-influencing therapies such as the treatment of cheilognathopalatoschisis in patients over 18 years old. Aesthetic issues influence subjective views of the therapeutic benefit, and it is unclear whether questions of current fashion or manifest efficacy predominate. A large-scale European multi-centre comparative study of therapies for this condition concentrated on analysis of the effects on skeletal growth. The only stringent variable proved to be the experience of the practitioner – in other words, the intrinsic evidence was found to be much more important than methodology. The conclusion in the British National Health Service was that there should be only a small number of treatment centres, each treating more than 20 children per year.

Strategies will no doubt have to be adapted in the future to problems amenable to them, in order to improve the quality of the results on which we base our activity. The latest Evidence-Based Dentistry Supplement to the British Dental Journal (1999) includes two reviews completed by the Cochrane Oral Health Group: "Orthodontic treatments for posterior crossbites" (Harrison, J. & Asby, D.) and, on the therapy of lichen ruber, "Interventions for treating oral lichen planus" (Chan, E., Thornhill, M. & Zakrzewska, J.).

The latter review evaluates the literature on the treatment of lichen ruber planus. A total of nine studies in four groups (cyclosporine, retinoids, steroids and phototherapy) are compared. The review is confined to these high-grade prospective randomized studies. Weak evidence for the efficacy of all methods was found, but no difference between them. It was concluded that further standardized, carefully selected studies were needed. If the non-randomized studies had also been thoroughly analysed, the important issue of the differences might also have been resolved.

9.8 Importance of EBM for quality assurance

There is no question that EBM methods also make an important contribution to quality assurance in dental work, in the sense that experts take the trouble to explore, evaluate and digest the literature to provide a basis for colleagues in dental practice, for appropriate statements and for continuing education. New academic disciplines are likely to be established, as the plethora of information accruing in scientific publications cannot be rated and integrated for the purposes of one's daily work without professional assistance. In this connection, the Cochrane Collaboration (cf. Antes & Linde, 1995), as an institution operating at international level, is surely important in the field of quality assurance. The enormous responsibility of compiling scientific systematic reviews falls to these groups, whose work ought there-

Table 9-6: Result of Medline searches for EBM and EBD		
Year	Evidence-based medicine	Evidence-based dentistry
	Number of publications	
1996	214	5
1997	604	5
1998	951	7
1999	866	8

fore to be recognized in academic circles as constituting a new scientific discipline.

Consideration of the literature on EBM (a simple Medline search – see Table 9-6) reveals an increasing proportion of evidence-based medicine citations. Based on titles in the field of evidence-based dentistry, the number of citations totals only 25. The subject has begun to feature in the dental literature too, albeit with a time lag.

9.9 Outlook

Good-quality studies based on EBM criteria are being conducted and will increasingly also influence clinical research strategies because they may help to validate the general conclusions drawn from them. In particular, clinical research and the handling of international research results will be crucially modified. However, this should not be seen as an isolated measure: what is needed is a multimodal, critical research approach involving validly underpinned decision-making aids to help practitioner and patient determine the appropriate treatment *on a scientific basis deemed valid at the time*. Yet being a doctor or dentist involves more than treating a patient in accordance with the latest discoveries of evidence-based medicine, and medicine is more than the sum of science and technology (cf. Diehl, 1999).

9.10 Literatur/References

ÄZQ, Zentralstelle der Deutschen Ärzteschaft zur Qualitätssicherung in der Medizin (Hrsg.): Leitlinien-In-Fo: das Leitlinien-Informations- und Fortbildungsprogramm der Ärztlichen Zentralstelle Qualitätssicherung. Schriftenreihe der Ärztlichen Zentralstelle Qualitätssicherung, Band 1. München 1999, 50

Antes, G., Linde, K.: Die Cochrane Collaboration; systematische Übersichten randomisierter klinischer Studien. Dt Ärztebl 92 (1995), B-224

Diehl, V.: Vortrag anlässlich der Eröffnung des Internisten-Kongresses, 1999

Egger, M., Zellweger, T., Antes, G.: Randomised trials in German-language journals. Lancet 347 (1996), 1047–1048

Evidence-based dentistry/Supplement to the British Dental Journal: Cochrane Oral Health Group, Completed reviews. 1 (1999) Heft 2/Juni 1999, 23

Kerschbaum, T.: Ergebnisorientierte Versorgung mit Kronen und Brücken. In: *Heidemann, D.* (Hrsg.): Zahnärztekalender 2000. München, 53–67

Meyer, R.: Culture based medicine: Landessitten und Therapierichtlinien. Dt Ärztebl 96 Heft 45 (1999), C-2084

Meyle, J.: Evidence based medicine (EBM) in der Parodontologie. In: *Heidemann, D.* (Hrsg.): Zahnärztekalender 2000. München, 33–44

Perleth, M.: Gegenwärtiger Stand der Evidenz-basierten Medizin. Z Allg Med 74 (1998), 450–454

Porzolt, F., Kunz, R.: Unterschiede zwischen Evidence-Based Medicine und konventionell bester Medizin. Medizinische Klinik 92 (1997), 567–569

Reich, E.: Evidenzbasierte Kariologie. In: *Heidemann, D.* (Hrsg.): Zahnärztekalender 2000. München, 1–32

Reinert, S., Krimmel, M.: Evidence based medicine in der Mund-Kiefer-Gesichtschirurgie. In: *Heidemann, D.* (Hrsg.): Zahnärztekalender 2000. München, 45–52

Sackett, D. L., Richardson, W. S., Rosenberg, W., Haynes, R. B.: Evidence-based Medicine. How to practice and teach EBM. New York (u. a.), 1997

10 EBM-Konzepte aus standespolitischer Sicht der Bundeszahnärztekammer – Anforderungen und Folgerungen

Peter Boehme, Bremen

Am Ende eines langen und intensiven Fortbildungstages haben sich neue Erkenntnisse und auch einige Kernaussagen herauskristallisiert. Es soll der Versuch unternommen werden, das Expertengespräch aus standespolitischer Sicht in sieben Punkten zusammenzufassen.

> **1. Die deutsche Zahnärzteschaft hat die Bedeutung der evidenz-basierten Zahnheilkunde erkannt und stellt sich dieser Aufgabe in enger Zusammenarbeit zwischen Wissenschaft und Praxis.**

Evidenz-basierte Medizin ist in der Medizin seit längerem etabliert. Die Zahnmedizin der Zukunft wird immer „medizinischer" werden. Über den Zusammenhang zwischen Zahnkrankheiten und Allgemeinkrankheiten gibt es neue Erkenntnisse. Zum Beispiel ist nachgewiesen, dass Zahnbetterkrankungen häufig mit Herz-/Kreislauferkrankungen korrespondieren. Immer mehr alte Menschen, die prothetisch versorgt werden müssen, weisen eine Multimorbidität auf. Die zahnmedizinische Versorgung ist in vielen Fällen ohne Kenntnisse der Psychosomatik nicht zufrieden stellend zu erbringen (z. B. bei Prothesenunverträglichkeiten). Daraus ergibt sich, dass die medizinische und die zahnmedizinische Forschung der Zukunft näher zusammenrücken werden. Es wird fließende Übergänge zwischen evidenzbasierter Medizin und evidenz-basierter Zahnheilkunde geben. Darüber hinaus wird die zahnmedizinische Forschung ihr wissenschaftliches Methodeninventar verbreitern und biostatistische und klinisch-epidemiologische Studienverfahren verstärkt einsetzen. Auch dadurch werden Erkenntnisse zu diagnostischen und/oder therapeutischen Verfahren auf einen neuen Level externer Evidenz gestellt werden.

> **2. Evidenz-basierte Zahnheilkunde ist zwar gegenwärtig ein Modethema, sie kann jedoch helfen, Therapieentscheidungen der Zukunft sicherer zu machen.**

Nur wenige Aussagen in der Zahnheilkunde sind bisher wissenschaftlich fundiert (8–15%, siehe hierzu auch Kapitel 6). Bei der Cochrane-Collaboration werden zurzeit aus der Zahnheilkunde nur Füllungsmaterialien und Prophylaxethemen bearbeitet. Weiter ist zu bedenken, dass nur mit wissenschaftlich fundierten Feststellungen die Aussagen bestimmter Gruppen, wie z. B. der Industrie, kommerzieller Gruppen, Patientenhilfeorganisationen, bestimmter zahnärztlicher Gruppen (biologische Zahnheilkunde) auf ihren Wahrheitsgehalt überprüft werden können. Die Aufgabe von evidenz-basierter Zahnheilkunde wird es sein, die Anliegen des Patienten in den Mittelpunkt der zahnärztlichen Therapieentscheidung zu stellen (siehe hierzu auch Kapitel 5). Die zahnärztliche Therapieentscheidung wird dort, wo wissenschaftlich fundierte Daten vorliegen, in Zukunft sicherer getroffen werden können. Allerdings wird die Evidenz immer nur ein Teil der Entscheidung sein können (siehe hierzu auch Kapitel 2).

Da sich das Wissen in unserer Zeit sehr schnell verändert, kann man evidenz-basierte Zahnheilkunde als „Update der Therapie-Software unter Qualitätsaspekten" bezeichnen. Die Grenzen von EBD liegen darin, dass wir durch sie für den individuellen Entscheidungsfall keine Vorgaben finden werden (siehe hierzu auch Kapitel 5).

> **3. Qualitätssicherung nimmt in der Zahnmedizin schon heute einen breiten Raum ein.**

Das Ziel aller qualitätssichernden Maßnahmen in der Zahnheilkunde ist der Erhalt oraler Strukturen des Patienten. Der Erhalt oraler Strukturen wird am besten gewährleistet durch die Hinwendung zu einer präventionsorientierten Zahnheilkunde. Dabei steht der eigenverantwortliche Patient (oral health self care) im Mittelpunkt der zahnärztlichen Bemühungen.

Es gibt heute schon eine ganze Reihe gesetzlicher Auflagen zur Qualitätssicherung, die durch das Gesundheitsstrukturgesetz 2000 leider im Sinne einer überbordenden Bürokratie nicht verbessert werden. Es besteht die begründete Gefahr, dass das oben genannte Ziel der Qualitätssicherung durch Erhebung und Zusammenführung überflüssiger Daten, kostenträchtiges Berichtswesen und externer Kontrollen aus den Augen verloren wird.

Es gibt in der Zahnmedizin eine sehr rege, freiwillige Fortbildung, die flächendeckend angeboten wird. Dort spielt das Thema EBM/EBD schon heute eine große Rolle. In über 200 zahnärztlichen Qualitätszirkeln (mit steigender Tendenz) werden wissenschaftliche Daten auf ihre Praktikabilität im Berufsalltag untersucht.

Bei Kammern und KZVen gibt es verschiedene Institutionen, die sich mit dem Thema Qualitätssicherung beschäftigen (z. B. Qualitätsbeauftragte, Tübinger Gutachtermodell, Wirtschaftlichkeitsprüfung u. a.).

Das Institut der Deutschen Zahnärzte (IDZ) hat mit seinen Mundgesundheitsstudien DMS I, II und DMS III den Beweis erbracht, dass sich die Mundgesundheit der deutschen Bevölkerung in den letzten zehn Jahren verbessert hat. Daran hat neben der allgemeinen Aufklärung und den verstärkten gruppenprophylaktischen Interventionen gewiss der zahnärztliche Berufsstand einen entscheidenden Anteil.

> **4. Der Ausschuss Qualitätssicherung der Bundeszahnärztekammer mit Beteiligung der KZBV und der DGZMK bearbeitet Fragen der evidenz-basierten Zahnheilkunde.**

Der Ausschuss sichtet und bewertet existierende Qualitätssicherungsmaßnahmen. Er initiiert neue Qualitätssicherungsmaßnahmen. Er hat eine „Leitlinie für Leitlinien" entwickelt und von den Vorständen verabschieden lassen, die eine Richtschnur für die Erarbeitung von Leitlinien der Zukunft darstellen soll. Hier gilt es, aus den Fehlern der Ärzteschaft mit einer Flut von Leitlinien unterschiedlicher Güteklasse zu lernen. Der Ausschuss Qualitätssicherung hat inzwischen zwei Pilotleitlinien in Auftrag gegeben. Dies sind die Leitlinie „Kariesprophylaxe mit Fluoriden" und die Leitlinie „Prävention und Intervention an Fissuren und Grübchen". Die Erarbeitung, Umsetzung und Evaluation von Leitlinien ist eine große Zukunftsaufgabe und kann nur durch Rückkopplung in Forschung und Praxis gelingen.

Brandaktuell ist die Nachricht, dass Bundeszahnärztekammer und Kassenzahnärztliche Bundesvereinigung vom Januar 2000 ab eine „Zahnärztliche Zentralstelle Qualitätssicherung" (zzq) als eigene Stabsstelle im Institut der Deutschen Zahnärzte eingerichtet haben. Dazu ist die Bereitstellung erheblicher finanzieller Mittel erforderlich. Das erfordert: Bei der Arbeit werden wir Prioritäten setzen müssen.

> **5. Wie sieht die zahnärztliche Standespolitik die Philosophie von evidenz-basierten Leitlinien?**

Leitlinien sollen für den Zahnarzt Entscheidungshilfen sein. Sie sollen ihm mehr Sicherheit bei Diagnose und Therapie geben.

Die Entscheidung ist der wichtigste Teil der zahnärztlichen Tätigkeit (siehe hierzu auch Kapitel 1). Befunderhebung und Dokumentation werden in Zukunft ein größeres Gewicht erhalten (siehe hierzu auch Kapitel 5).

Leitlinien werden einen neuen Forschungsbedarf aufzeigen. Bei schwierigen Problemen müssen verfeinerte Methoden angewendet werden (siehe hierzu auch Kapitel 3). Evidenz-basierte Medizin/evidenz-basierte Zahnheilkunde kostet Geld, das von der Gesellschaft aufgebracht werden muss.

Die Leitlinie kann dem einzelnen Zahnarzt nur einen Handlungskorridor zeigen. Sie muss als externe Evidenz mit der individuellen klinischen Erfahrung des Zahnarztes verbunden werden. Die subjektive Patientensicht ist ein eigenständiger Faktor bei allen Diagnose- und Therapiefragen. Der kommunikativen Evidenz ist daher die pragmatische Evidenz im Praxisalltag entgegenzustellen (siehe hierzu auch Kapitel 4).

Extrem wichtig ist deshalb die Praktikabilität von Leitlinien und ihre Implementation in den Versorgungsalltag (siehe hierzu auch Kapitel 2).

Leitlinien können die autoritäre Feststellung auf unbekannter Wissensbasis sein oder auf strukturierten Erkenntnissen beruhen (siehe hierzu auch Kapitel 5). Der Evidenz-Grad ist daher offen zu legen.

Leitlinien sind keine Kassen-Richtlinien (siehe hierzu auch Kapitel 6). Sie beruhen auf wissenschaftlich fundierten fachlichen Aussagen. Versicherungstechnische Grenzen zahnmedizinischer Versorgungssysteme müssen auf einer anderen Ebene ausgehandelt werden.

Leitlinien müssen zur Anwendung ständig re-evaluiert werden und sind nach dem jeweiligen Wissensstand regelmäßig zu aktualisieren.

Die mit EBM/EBD verbundenen Ängste und Hoffnungen beziehen sich auf die Therapieentscheidungen (siehe hierzu auch Kapitel 5). Da eine systematische Erhebung aller entscheidungsrelevanten wissenschaftlichen Daten niemals stattfinden wird, kann evidenz-basierte Zahnheilkunde nur einige Teilchen zu dem großen Puzzlespiel bei der Entscheidungsfindung in der Praxis beitragen. Eine Gefahr von Therapiestandards durch EBM/EBD in der Zahnheilkunde ist zurzeit unbegründet.

> **6. EBM bzw. EBD hat Einfluss auf Systemfragen der gesundheitlichen Versorgung.**

EBM/EBD heißt keineswegs automatisch billiger, sondern kann, wenn neue Verfahren kostenaufwendiger sind, auch teurer sein. Kosten-Nutzendiskussionen, wie sie in der Politik geführt werden, können nicht durch EBM/EBD ersetzt werden. Innerhalb der gesetzlichen Krankenversicherung sind z. B. der medizinische Nutzen, die medizinische Notwendigkeit und die Wirtschaftlichkeit von Maßnahmen drei eigenständige Parameter der versorgungspolitischen Entscheidung. Aber wo immer ein ökonomischer Vergleich zwischen verschiedenen gleich evidenten Behandlungsmethoden möglich ist, ist die preiswertere Methode auch die effizientere.

Evidenz-basierte Medizin hinkt dem Fortschritt hinterher. Schnelle Entwicklungen (wie z. B. Vector, Composites, Bonder) können noch nicht evidenz-basiert sein. Klinische Langzeituntersuchungen kommen oft zu spät, weil sich Material und Methoden in unserer Zeit rasant schnell weiterentwickeln. Auch ist die Validität der durch EBD erhobenen Daten in verschiedenen Untersuchungen oft unterschiedlich und schwer zu vergleichen (siehe hierzu auch Kapitel 7).

Einer evidenz-basierten Zahnheilkunde werden daher auch in Zukunft Grenzen gesetzt sein. Eine große Sorge besteht darin, dass Leitlinien zwar nicht juristisch, aber normativ verbindlich sein können (siehe hierzu auch Kapitel 3). Eine Mutation von Leitlinien zu Richtlinien wäre aber für den EBM-Gedanken im Grunde tödlich. EBM/EBD kann für die Krankenkassen keine Planungsgröße zur Kostenkontrolle sein.

Zurzeit sind die forensischen Folgen von EBM/EBD allerdings noch nicht absehbar.

Auch in Zukunft wird die Zahnheilkunde mit Unsicherheiten leben müssen. Evidenz bezieht sich immer nur auf den jetzigen Zeitpunkt.

Positive Folgen von EBM/EBD werden (siehe hierzu auch Kapitel 5) allerdings sein:

– die Standardisierung der zahnmedizinischen Forschung und

– ein Bedeutungsgewinn von wissenschaftlichen Begründungen bei klinischen Entscheidungen.

> **7. EBM bzw. EBD muss im Zusammenhang mit der allgemeinen Gesundheitspolitik gesehen werden.**

– EBM/EBD wird das Arzt-Patienten-Verhältnis verändern in Richtung mehr Kommunikation, mehr Aufklärungsbedarf usw.
– EBM/EBD wird auch das Verhältnis zwischen medizinischer Wissenschaft und medizinischer Praxis verändern (mehr Austausch, vielleicht auch mehr Konflikte).
– EBM/EBD wird im Zeitalter der elektronischen Medien zu einer „kognitiven Globalisierung" des medizinischen Wissens führen. Die Ausbreitung des Wissens wird mit einer viel größeren Geschwindigkeit als früher erzielt werden.
– EBM/EBD wird zunehmend auch das Kosten-Nutzen-Abwägen in der Medizin beeinflussen und langfristig wohl auch die gesellschaftlichen Gesundheitsvorstellungen mit prägen. Da sich viele Parameter (wie z. B. die dentofaziale Ästhetik, die subjektive Patientenzufriedenheit o. ä.) nicht in EBM/EBD-Untersuchungen ausdrücken lassen, wird es immer eine individuelle Seite des Arzt-Patienten-Verhältnisses geben, die über Erfolg oder Misserfolg der Behandlung entscheidet.
– EBM/EBD läuft Gefahr, zu eng gesehen zu werden. Auch interdisziplinäre

Forschungsergebnisse müssen aufgenommen werden, z. B. kulturelle Anteile im Verständnis von Einzelkrankheiten.
– EBM/EBD ist kein Selbstzweck. Die so gewonnenen Erkenntnisse müssen von Praktikern der medizinischen Versorgung auf ihren Erkenntnisbeitrag befragt werden können. Qualitätszirkel sind hier ein höchst nützliches Medium.
– EBM/EBD sollte nicht zu hoch bewertet werden. Sie kann Gesundheitspolitik niemals ersetzen. Vielmehr wird sich die Gesundheitspolitik zukünftig verstärkt dem Entscheidungsdruck stellen müssen, der durch evidenz-basiertes Wissen zu Fragen der medizinischen Diagnostik und Therapie zusätzlich ausgelöst wird.

Damit schließt sich der Kreis, wobei jedoch noch auf einen Satz hingewiesen werden soll, der überall im Leben gilt und nur bei den Heilberufen zurzeit durch die staatliche Gesundheitspolitik aufgehoben sein soll: Qualität hat ihren Preis.

10 EBM concepts from the point of view of the profession as represented by the Bundeszahnärztekammer [German Dental Association] – requirements and conclusions

Peter Boehme, Bremen

At the end of a long and concentrated day of further study, new realizations and also a few central propositions have emerged. This paper attempts to summarize the expert colloquium in seven points as seen by the profession.

> 1. The dental profession in Germany has recognized the importance of evidence-based dentistry, which it is espousing by a process of close collaboration between science and practice.

Evidence-based medicine already has a fairly long tradition in the medical field. The dentistry of the future will become increasingly "medical". New discoveries have been made about the connection between dental pathology and general diseases. For example, pathology of the tooth-supporting tissues has been demonstrated to correlate with cardiovascular diseases. More and more older people requiring dental prostheses exhibit multimorbidity. Satisfactory dental care can often not be provided without a knowledge of psychosomatic medicine (e.g. in cases of prosthetic intolerance). In consequence, medical and dental research will move closer together in the future. The boundary between evidence-based medicine and evidence-based dentistry will become blurred. In addition, dental research will broaden its inventory of scientific methods and resort increasingly to biostatic study techniques and those of clinical epidemiology. This too will contribute to placing knowledge of diagnostic and/or therapeutic methods on a new footing of external evidence.

> 2. Evidence-based dentistry is not merely fashionable but really can help to make future decisions on therapy more certain.

Not very many propositions in the dental field are at present supported by scientific evidence (8–15% of the total, according to chapter 6). Current work in the dental field in the Cochrane Collaboration relates only to filling materials and matters of prophylaxis. Furthermore, the truth of the claims of certain groups – such as industry, commercial undertakings, patient-help organizations and some dental groups (biological dentistry) – can be verified only by scientifically based findings. Evidence-based dentistry will have the task of placing patients' wishes at the focus of decisions on dental therapy (see chapter 5). The making of these therapeutic decisions will be more certain in the future where scientifically based data are available. However, evidence will always remain only a part of the decision-making process (see chapter 2).

Owing to the current rapid rate of change in knowledge, evidence-based dentistry can be described as an "update of therapy software in quality terms" (see chapter 5). The limits of EBD lie in the fact that it will not lay down a course of action for us in any individual decision situation, as Professor Walther also notes in his chapter.

3. Quality assurance already plays an important part in many fields of dentistry today.

The aim of all quality assurance measures in dentistry is the preservation of the patient's oral structures. This goal can best be achieved by the adoption of a form of dentistry oriented towards prevention. Here the dentist's primary objective will be the assumption of responsibility by the patient himself (oral health self-care).

A whole series of legal precepts on quality assurance are already in force in Germany, and unfortunately the Health Structure Law 2000 does nothing to stem the flood tide of bureaucracy. There is reason to fear that the above aim of quality assurance will be lost sight of through the recording and collation of superfluous data, expensive reporting and external inspections.

A highly active system of voluntary continuing education covering the entire country exists in the dental field. The subject of EBM/EBD already plays a major part in it today. The practical applicability of scientific data to the daily exercise of the profession is being examined in over 200 dental quality circles (whose number is constantly increasing).

Various institutions within the professional dental organizations (Chambers and KZVs [Associations of Sick Fund Dentists]) are engaged on quality assurance issues – for example, quality officers, the Tübingen Expert Reporting Model, verification of economic efficiency, and so on.

Through its oral health studies (DMS I, II and III), the Institute of German Dentists (IDZ) has shown that the German population's oral health has improved in the last ten years. This is surely due in no small measure to the efforts of the dental profession, as well as to general information campaigns and the intensification of interventions in the field of group prophylaxis.

> **4. The Quality Assurance Committee of the BZÄK [German Dental Association], with the participation of the KZBV [Federal Authority for Dental Care] and the DGZMK [German Society of Dentistry and Oral Medicine], is working on evidence-based dentistry issues.**

The Committee scrutinizes and assesses existing quality assurance measures and initiates new ones. It has developed a "Guideline for Guidelines", intended as a master guide for drafting the guidelines of the future, which was adopted by the relevant executive bodies. The aim is to learn from the mistakes of the medical profession, which has a plethora of guidelines of varying quality. The Quality Assurance Committee has since commissioned two pilot guidelines, one on "caries prophylaxis with fluorides" and the other on the "prevention and treatment of pits and fissures". The drafting, implementation and evaluation of guidelines is a major task for the future and can succeed only through feedback in research and practice.

The very latest news is that the German Dental Association and the Federal Authority for Dental Care have established the "Agency for Quality in Dentistry" (known by its German initials zzq), to operate as an internal staff body within the Institute of German Dentists with effect from January 2000. This will call for the provision of substantial funds, so that priorities will have to be set for its work.

> **5. What is the dental profession's view of the philosophy of evidence-based guidelines?**

Guidelines are intended as aids to decision-making for the dentist, providing him or her with more certainty in diagnosis and therapy.

Decision-making is the most important component of dental activity (see chapter 1). In the future more emphasis will be placed on the recording of findings and on documentation (see chapter 5).

Guidelines will indicate where new research is needed. More sophisticated methods will be necessary for difficult problems (see chapter 3). Evidence-based medicine and evidence-based dentistry cost money, which will have to be provided by society.

A guideline can do no more than show the individual dentist a corridor for action. As external evidence, it must be combined with the dentist's individual clinical experience. The subjective view of the patient is a factor in its own right in all matters of diagnosis and therapy. For this reason the pragmatic evidence must be compared with the communicative evidence in the course of the dentist's daily practice (see chapter 4).

The practicability of guidelines and their implementation in the routine treatment situation are therefore extremely important (see chapter 2).

Guidelines may be authoritarian statements resting on an unknown foundation or they may be based on structured evidence (see chapter 5). Hence the degree of evidence must be specified.

Guidelines are not sick fund directives (see chapter 6). They are supported by scientific evidence. Insurance-related issues and their boundaries regarding dental care systems must be negotiated on a different level.

Guidelines must be constantly re-evaluated for the purpose of application and must be regularly updated in accordance with the latest state of the art.

The anxieties and hopes associated with EBM/EBD concern therapeutic decisions (see chapter 5). Since it will never be possible to record all the scientific data relevant to decision-making, evidence-based dentistry will be able to contribute only a few pieces to the huge jigsaw puzzle of decision-making in clinical practice. There is at present no danger of therapy standards being set by EBM/EBD in dentistry.

6. EBM and EBD affect system policy issues in health care.

EBM/EBD is not automatically synonymous with lower cost; where new techniques are dearer, it may actually be more expensive. Cost-benefit debate as in the political sphere cannot be replaced by EBM/EBD. Within the legal system of health insurance, the medical benefit, the medical need and the economic aspects of measures are three autonomous parameters of care-policy decision-making. Wherever an economic comparison between different treatment methods supported by equal degrees of evidence is possible, however, the cheaper method will be the more efficient.

Evidence-based medicine lags behind progress. Fast-developing fields, e.g. regarding dental materials (such as Vector, composites and bonding agents), cannot yet be evidence-based. Long-term clinical studies often come too late owing to today's enormous pace of development in materials and methods. Moreover, the degree of validity of the data recorded by EBD in different studies is often variable, so that the data are not readily comparable (see chapter 7).

Hence limits will apply to an evidence-based dentistry in the future as they do today. A major concern is that guidelines, while not binding legally, may be so on the normative level (see chapter 3). However, if guidelines were to become directives, that would be fatal to the idea of EBM. EBM/EBD cannot be used by the health insurance funds as a planning parameter for cost control.

At present, though, the forensic consequences of EBM/EBD cannot be foreseen.

Dentistry will have to go on living with uncertainty in the future. Evidence always relates only to the present.

But EBM/EBD will have the following positive consequences (see chapter 5):

– standardization of dental research,

– increased significance of scientific evidence in clinical decision-making.

7. EBM and EBD must be seen in the context of overall health policy.

– EBM/EBD will change the doctor-patient relationship in the direction of more communication, a greater need for patient information, etc.
– EBM/EBD will also alter the relationship between medical science and medical practice (more reciprocal contact and perhaps also more conflicts).
– EBM/EBD will, in the age of the electronic media, lead to a "cognitive globalization" of medical knowledge. Information will be disseminated much more quickly than in the past.
– EBM/EBD will also increasingly influence the weighing of costs against benefits in medicine and will, in the long term, no doubt also contribute to determining social policy on health issues. Since many parameters (e.g. dentofacial aesthetics, subjective patient satisfaction and the like) cannot be expressed in EBM/EBD reviews, there will always be an individual side to the doctor-patient relationship that will determine the success or failure of the treatment.
– EBM/EBD risks being seen too narrowly. Interdisciplinary research results must be included in its remit – e.g. cultural aspects in the understanding of individual disease entities.
– EBM/EBD is not an end in itself. It must be possible for medical practitioners to question its results in terms of their contribution to knowledge. Quality circles are a very valuable institution for this purpose.
– EBM/EBD should not be overrated. It can never replace health policy. Instead, health policy will in the future have to submit to the increased pressure on decision-making that will result from evidence-based knowledge in matters of medical diagnosis and therapy.

That, then, completes the circle, but a principle should not be forgotten that governs all aspects of life and – due to the government's health policy – is currently supposed to be inapplicable only in the healing professions: quality has its price.

11 Verzeichnis der Autoren/List of Contributors

Dr. med. dent. Peter Boehme
Vorstandsmitglied der Bundeszahnärztekammer
Köln – Bremen

Professor Dr. med. dent. Michael Heners
Akademie für Zahnärztliche Fortbildung Karlsruhe
Karlsruhe

Professor Dr. med. Jörg Michael Herrmann
Reha-Klinik Glotterbad
Glottertal

Professor Dr. med. dent. Thomas Kerschbaum
Zentrum für Zahn-, Mund- und Kieferheilkunde der Universität zu Köln
Vorklinische Zahnheilkunde
Köln

Professor Dr. med. dent. Jörg Meyle
Med. Zentrum für Zahn-, Mund- und Kieferheilkunde
am Klinikum der Justus-Liebig-Universität Gießen
Abteilung Parodontologie
Gießen

Dr. disc. pol. Wolfgang Micheelis
Institut der Deutschen Zahnärzte
Köln

Dr. med. Matthias Perleth, M.S.P.
Abt. Epidemiologie, Sozialmedizin und Gesundheitssystemforschung
Medizinische Hochschule Hannover
Hannover

Professor Dr. med. dent. Elmar Reich
Abt. Parodontologie und Zahnerhaltung
Universität Homburg
Homburg an der Saar

Professor Dr. Derek Richards, BDS, MSc, DDPH, FDS (DPH)
Centre for Evidence-based Dentistry, Institute of Health Sciences
Oxford

Professor Dr. med. Thure von Uexküll
Freiburg

Professor Dr. med. Dr. med. dent. Wilfried Wagner
Deutsche Gesellschaft für Zahn-, Mund- und Kieferheilkunde
Johannes Gutenberg-Universität
Klinik für Mund-, Kiefer- und Gesichtschirurgie
Mainz

Professor Dr. med. dent. Winfried Walther
Akademie für Zahnärztliche Fortbildung Karlsruhe
Karlsruhe

12 Verzeichnis der Abbildungen und Tabellen

Abbildungen

Abbildung 1-1: Etappen in der Wissenschaftlichkeit von Medizin und Zahnheilkunde
Abbildung 1-2: Das Prinzip der induktiv-deduktiven Erkenntnis
Abbildung 1-3: Parameter der zahnärztlichen Therapie und Therapieentscheidung
Abbildung 2-1: Faktoren, die die Behandlungsentscheidung beeinflussen
Abbildung 2-2: Innovationsumweg
Abbildung 2-3: Einschätzung der aktuellen Evidenz-Basis für zahnärztliche Maßnahmen
Abbildung 2-4: Angestrebte Zielsetzung für die Evidenz-Basis zahnärztlicher Maßnahmen
Abbildung 3-1: Zusammenhang zwischen Wirksamkeit und Instrumenten zum Nachweis der Wirksamkeit
Abbildung 3-2: Logo der Cochrane Collaboration
Abbildung 3-3: Risikoverteilung in verschiedenen Studien
Abbildung 3-4: „Effectiveness Domain"
Abbildung 5-1: Behandlungsfall mit ästhetischer Problematik
Abbildung 5-2: Modell Befund – Therapie
Abbildung 5-3: Entscheidungsmodell „Patientenanliegen – Befund – Therapeutische Software"
Abbildung 5-4: Patientenorientiertes Entscheidungsmodell
Abbildung 5-5: Die evidenz-basierte Zahnmedizin ist im Rahmen des patientenorientierten Entscheidungsmodells der empirischen Wissensbasis des Arztes zuzuordnen
Abbildung 5-6: Überlebenskurven als Ergebnis einer klinischen Fragestellung zum Erfolg vergleichbarer Therapien
Abbildung 6-1: Häufigkeit von Zahnersatz in Prozent
Abbildung 6-2: Behandlungsalternativen bei einer Frontzahnlücke (Adhäsivbrücke, konventionelle Brücke, Einzelimplantat, kieferorthopädischer Lückenschluss, partielle Prothese, UDA-Brücken)
Abbildung 6-3: Prothetische Alternativen zur Versorgung von Freiendsituationen
Abbildung 7-1: Sensivität und Spezifität verschiedener Methoden zur Diagnose der Okklusalkaries

Abbildung 7-2: Durchschnittliche Fähigkeit (Dz) verschiedener diagnostischer Methoden für die Diagnose der Approximalkaries
Abbildung 7-3: Anteil Versiegelungen an Molaren bayerischer Kinder
Abbildung 7-4: Lebensdauer von Restaurationen

Tabellen

Tabelle 2-1: Adäquanz von Studiendesigns
Tabelle 2-2: Evidenz-Basis in der Zahnheilkunde
Tabelle 2-3: Fehler im Studiendesign
Tabelle 3-1: Komponenten der systematischen Übersicht
Tabelle 3-2: Unterschiede zwischen narrativen und systematischen Übersichten
Tabelle 5-1: Methodische Fragestellung zur Untersuchung einer veröffentlichten Meta-Studie
Tabelle 6-1: Zahnersatz in mittleren und höheren Altersstufen
Tabelle 6-2: Kosten und mittlere Überlebensdauer verschiedener prothetischer Therapiemittel
Tabelle 6-3: Langzeitergebnisse zum Überleben von Kronen und Brücken
Tabelle 6-4: Langzeitergebnisse zum Überleben von Pfeilerzähnen
Tabelle 6-5: Anzahl DGZMK Statements in zahnmedizinischen Fachgebieten
Tabelle 7-1: Konsensus-Konferenz der CDA – Schlussfolgerungen zur täglichen Fluoridanwendung
Tabelle 8-1: Vereinfachtes Schema des Behandlungsablaufes bei adulter Parodontitis im Vergleich zum bestehenden PAR-Vertrag
Tabelle 8-2: Auswahl klinischer Vergleichsstudien zur Effizienz der subgingivalen Wurzeloberflächenreinigung (Deep Scaling)
Tabelle 8-3: Verfahren der Parodontalchirurgie zur Behandlung von entzündungsbedingten Defekten
Tabelle 9-1: Einteilung der Evidenzstärke nach AHCPR
Tabelle 9-2: Forschungsstrategie (begrenzende Fachprobleme)
Tabelle 9-3: Traditionelle und künftige Forschungsstrategie
Tabelle 9-4: Studiendesignbildungen
Tabelle 9-5: Priorisierungsliste
Tabelle 9-6: Ergebnis von Medline-Recherchen zu EBM und EBD

12 List of Figures and Tables

Figures

Figure 1-1: Stages in the evolution of the scientific status of medicine and dentistry
Figure 1-2: Epistemological principle of induction and deduction
Figure 1-3: Parameters of dental therapy and therapeutic decision-making
Figure 2-1: Influences on decisions
Figure 2-2: Innovation bypass
Figure 2-3: Estimate of the current position of the evidence-base of dental interventions
Figure 2-4: Future aim for the evidence-base of dental interventions
Figure 3-1: Relation of effectiveness and instruments for its demonstration
Figure 3-2: Logo of the Cochrane Collaboration
Figure 3-3: Risk distribution in various studies
Figure 3-4: "Effectiveness domain"
Figure 5-1: A clinical case involving aesthetic considerations
Figure 5-2: Findings-therapy model
Figure 5-3: Decision model based on "patient's wishes – findings – therapeutic software"
Figure 5-4: Patient-oriented decision model
Figure 5-5: In the patient-oriented decision model, evidence-based dentistry must be assigned to the dentist's empirical knowledge base
Figure 5-6: Survival curves resulting from a clinical question about the results of comparable therapies
Figure 6-1: Frequency of dental prostheses
Figure 6-2: Treatment options for an anterior tooth edentulous space (adhesive bridge, conventional bridge, single implant, orthodontic space closure, partial prosthesis, UDA bridge)
Figure 6-3: Prosthetic options for free-end situations
Figure 7-1: Sensitivity and specificity of different diagnostic methods for occlusal caries
Figure 7-2: Average effectiveness (Dz) of different diagnostic techniques for approximal caries
Figure 7-3: Percentage sealed molars in Bavarian children
Figure 7-4: Longevity of restorations

Tables

Table 2-1: Appropriate study designs
Table 2-2: The evidence-base for oral health
Table 2-3: Errors in study design
Table 3-1: Components of a systematic review
Table 3-2: Differences between narrative and systematic reviews
Table 5-1: Methodological questions for examining a published meta-study
Table 6-1: Prostheses in middle-aged and older subjects
Table 6-2: Cost and average survival period of different forms of prosthetic appliances
Table 6-3: Survival of crowns and bridges – long-term results
Table 6-4: Survival of abutment teeth – long-term results
Table 6-5: Numbers of DGZMK Statements in dental specialties
Table 7-1: Consensus Conference of the Canadian Dental Association – conclusion on daily fluoride use
Table 8-1: Simplified breakdown of treatment sequence for adult periodontitis vs existing periodontology contract
Table 8-2: Selection of comparative clinical trials on the efficacy of subgingival root surface cleaning (deep scaling)
Table 8-3: Periodontal surgical procedures for the treatment of defects due to inflammation
Table 9-1: Grading of evidence by the AHCPR
Table 9-2: Research strategy (limitation to specific issues)
Table 9-3: Traditional and future research strategies
Table 9-4: Types of study design
Table 9-5: Priority list
Table 9-6: Result of Medline searches for EBM and EBD

Veröffentlichungen des Instituts der Deutschen Zahnärzte

Stand: März 2000

Materialienreihe

Amalgam – Pro und Contra. Gutachten – Referate – Statements – Diskussion. Wissenschaftliche Bearbeitung und Kommentierung von G. Knolle, IDZ-Materialienreihe Bd. 1, 3. erweiterte Aufl., ISBN 3-7691-7830-0, Deutscher Ärzte-Verlag, 1992

Parodontalgesundheit der Hamburger Bevölkerung. Epidemiologische Ergebnisse einer CPITN-Untersuchung. G. Ahrens/J. Bauch/K.-A. Bublitz/ I. Neuhaus, IDZ-Materialienreihe Bd. 2, ISBN 3-7691-7812-2, Deutscher Ärzte-Verlag, 1988

Zahnarzt und Praxiscomputer. Ergebnisse einer empirischen Erhebung. S. Becker/F. W. Wilker, unter Mitarbeit von W. Micheelis, IDZ-Materialienreihe Bd. 3, ISBN 3-7691-7813-0, Deutscher Ärzte-Verlag, 1988

Der Zahnarzt im Blickfeld der Ergonomie. Eine Analyse zahnärztlicher Arbeitshaltungen. W. Rohmert/J. Mainzer/P. Zipp, IDZ-Materialienreihe Bd. 4, 2. unveränderte Aufl., ISBN 3-7691-7814-9, Deutscher Ärzte-Verlag, 1988

Möglichkeiten und Auswirkungen der Förderung der Zahnprophylaxe und Zahnerhaltung durch Bonussysteme. M. Schneider, IDZ-Materialienreihe Bd. 5, ISBN 3-7691-7815-7, Deutscher Ärzte-Verlag, 1988

Mundgesundheitsberatung in der Zahnarztpraxis. T. Schneller/D. Mittermeier/D. Schulte am Hülse/W. Micheelis, IDZ-Materialienreihe Bd. 6, ISBN 3-7691-7817-3, Deutscher Ärzte-Verlag, 1990

Aspekte zahnärztlicher Leistungsbewertung aus arbeitswissenschaftlicher Sicht. M. Essmat/W. Micheelis/G. Rennenberg, IDZ-Materialienreihe Bd. 7, ISBN 3-7691-7819-X, Deutscher Ärzte-Verlag, 1990

Wirtschaftszweig Zahnärztliche Versorgung. E. Helmstädter, IDZ-Materialienreihe Bd. 8, ISBN 3-7691-7821-1, Deutscher Ärzte-Verlag, 1990

Bedarf an Zahnärzten bis zum Jahre 2010. E. Becker/F.-M. Niemann/ J. G. Brecht/F. Beske, IDZ-Materialienreihe Bd. 9, ISBN 3-7691-7823-8, Deutscher Ärzte-Verlag, 1990

Der Praxiscomputer als Arbeitsmittel. Prüfsteine und Erfahrungen. M. Hildmann, unter Mitarbeit von W. Micheelis, IDZ-Materialienreihe Bd. 10, ISBN 3-7691-7824-6, Deutscher Ärzte-Verlag, 1991

Mundgesundheitszustand und -verhalten in der Bundesrepublik Deutschland. Ergebnisse des nationalen IDZ-Survey 1989. Gesamtbearbeitung: W. Micheelis, J. Bauch, mit Beiträgen von J. Bauch/P. Dünninger/ R. Eder-Debye/J. Einwag/J. Hoeltz/K. Keß/R. Koch/W. Micheelis/R. Naujoks/ K. Pieper/E. Reich/E. Witt, IDZ-Materialienreihe Bd. 11.1, ISBN 3-7691-7825-4, Deutscher Ärzte-Verlag, 1991

Oral Health in Germany: Diagnostic Criteria and Data Recording Manual. Instructions for examination and documentation of oral health status. – With an appendix of the sociological survey instruments for the assessment of oral health attitudes and behavior. J. Einwag/K. Keß/E. Reich, IDZ-Materialienreihe Bd. 11.2, ISBN 3-7691-7826-2, Deutscher Ärzte-Verlag, 1992

Mundgesundheitszustand und -verhalten in Ostdeutschland. Ergebnisse des IDZ-Ergänzungssurvey 1992. Gesamtbearbeitung: W. Micheelis, J. Bauch, mit Beiträgen von J. Bauch/A. Borutta/J. Einwag/J. Hoeltz/W. Micheelis/P. Potthoff/E. Reich/H. Stechemesser, IDZ-Materialienreihe Bd. 11.3, ISBN 3-7691-7834-3, Deutscher Ärzte-Verlag, 1993

Risikogruppenprofile bei Karies und Parodontitis. Statistische Vertiefungsanalysen der Mundgesundheitsstudien des IDZ von 1989 und 1992. Gesamtbearbeitung: W. Micheelis, E. Schroeder, mit Beiträgen von J. Einwag/W. Micheelis/P. Potthoff/E. Reich/E. Schroeder, IDZ-Materialienreihe Bd. 11.4, ISBN 3-7691-7839-4, Deutscher Ärzte-Verlag, 1996

Psychologische Aspekte bei der zahnprothetischen Versorgung. Eine Untersuchung zum Compliance-Verhalten von Prothesenträgern. T. Schneller/R. Bauer/W. Micheelis, IDZ-Materialienreihe Bd. 12, 2. unveränderte Aufl., ISBN 3-7691-7829-7, Deutscher Ärzte-Verlag, 1992

Gruppen- und Individualprophylaxe in der Zahnmedizin. Ein Handbuch für die prophylaktische Arbeit in Kindergarten, Schule und Zahnarztpraxis. Gesamtbearbeitung: N. Bartsch, J. Bauch, mit Beiträgen von N. Bartsch/ J. Bauch/K. Dittrich/G. Eberle/J. Einwag/H. Feser/K.-D. Hellwege/E. H. Hörschelmann/K. G. König/C. Leitzmann/F. Magri/J. Margraf-Stiksrud/W. Micheelis/H. Pantke/E. Reihlen/R. Roehl/F. Römer/H. P. Rosemeier/T. Schneller, IDZ-Materialienreihe Bd. 13, ISBN 3-7691-7829-9, Deutscher-Ärzte-Verlag, 1992

Betriebswirtschaftliche Entscheidungshilfen durch den Praxiscomputer. E. Knappe/V. Laine/P. Klein/S. Schmitz, IDZ-Materialienreihe Bd. 14, ISBN 3-7691-7831-9, Deutscher Ärzte-Verlag, 1992

Qualitätssicherung in der zahnmedizinischen Versorgung. Weißbuch. J. Bauch/J. Becker/E.-A. Behne/B. Bergmann-Krauss/P. Boehme/C. Boldt/ K. Bößmann/K. Budde/D. Buhtz/H.-J. Gronemeyer/K. Kimmel/H.-P. Küchenmeister/W. Micheelis/P. J. Müller/T. Muschallik/C.-T. Plöger/M. Schneider/ H. Spranger/M. Steudle/B. Tiemann/J. Viohl/K. Walther/W. Walther/J. Weitkamp/P. Witzel, IDZ-Materialienreihe Bd. 15, 2. Aufl., ISBN 3-7691-7837-8, Deutscher Ärzte-Verlag, 1995

Prophylaxe ein Leben lang. Ein lebensbegleitendes oralprophylaktisches Betreuungskonzept. Gesamtbearbeitung: J. Bauch, mit Beiträgen von N. Bartsch/J. Einwag/H.-J. Gülzow/G. Johnke/W. Kollmann/L. Laurisch/J. Magraf-Stiksrud/T. Schneller/K.-P. Wefers, IDZ-Materialienreihe Bd. 16, 2. unveränderte Aufl., ISBN 3-7691-7844-0, Deutscher Ärzte-Verlag, 1998

Streß bei Zahnärzten. Ch. von Quast, IDZ-Materialienreihe Bd. 17, ISBN 3-7691-7840-8, Deutscher Ärzte-Verlag, 1996

Zahnärztliche Qualitätszirkel. Grundlagen und Ergebnisse eines Modellversuches. W. Micheelis/W. Walther/J. Szecsenyi, IDZ-Materialienreihe Bd. 18, 2. unveränderte Aufl., ISBN 3-7691-7846-7, Deutscher Ärzte-Verlag, 1998

Hygiene in der Zahnarztpraxis. Ergebnisse einer Pilotstudie zu den betriebswirtschaftlichen Kosten. V. P. Meyer/D. Buhtz, IDZ-Materialienreihe Bd. 19, ISBN 3-7691-7842-4, Deutscher Ärzte-Verlag, 1998

Amalgam im Spiegel kritischer Auseinandersetzungen. Interdisziplinäre Stellungnahmen zum „Kieler Amalgam-Gutachten". S. Halbach, R. Hickel, H. Meiners, K. Ott, F. X. Reichl, R. Schiele, G. Schmalz, H. J. Staehle, IDZ-Materialienreihe Bd. 20, ISBN 3-7691-7847-5, Deutscher Ärzte-Verlag, 1999

Dritte Deutsche Mundgesundheitsstudie (DMS III). Ergebnisse, Trends und Problemanalysen auf der Grundlage bevölkerungsrepräsentativer Stichproben in Deutschland 1997. Gesamtbearbeitung: W. Micheelis, E. Reich, mit Beiträgen von R. Heinrich/M. John/E. Lenz/W. Micheelis/P. Potthoff/E. Reich/P. A. Reichart/U. Schiffner/E. Schroeder/I. von Törne/K.-P. Wefers, IDZ-Materialienreihe Bd. 21, ISBN 3-7691-7848-3, Deutscher Ärzte-Verlag, 1999

Ökonomische Effekte der Individualprophylaxe. Dokumentation eines computergestützten Simulationsmodells. Ralpf Kaufhold, Peter Biene-Dietrich, Uwe Hofmann, Wolfgang Micheelis, Lothar Scheibe, Markus Schneider, IDZ-Materialienreihe Bd. 22, ISBN 3-934280-14-5, Deutscher Zahnärzte Verlag, 1999

Broschürenreihe

Zur medizinischen Bedeutung der zahnärztlichen Therapie mit festsitzendem Zahnersatz (Kronen und Brücken) im Rahmen der Versorgung. T. Kerschbaum, IDZ-Broschürenreihe Bd. 1, ISBN 3-7691-7816-5, Deutscher Ärzte-Verlag, 1988

Zum Stand der EDV-Anwendung in der Zahnarztpraxis. Ergebnisse eines Symposions. IDZ-Broschürenreihe Bd. 2, ISBN 3-7691-7818-1, Deutscher Ärzte-Verlag, 1989

Mundgesundheit in der Bundesrepublik Deutschland. Ausgewählte Ergebnisse einer bevölkerungsrepräsentativen Erhebung des Mundgesundheitszustandes und -verhaltens in der Bundesrepublik Deutschland. IDZ-Broschürenreihe Bd. 3, ISBN 3-7691-7822-X, Deutscher Ärzte-Verlag, 1990

Interprofessionelle Zusammenarbeit in der zahnärztlichen Versorgung. Interprofessional Cooperation in Dental Care. Dokumentation – Documentation FDI-Symposium Berlin, September 1992. IDZ-Broschürenreihe Bd. 4, ISBN 3-7691-7833-5, Deutscher Ärzte-Verlag, 1993

Sonderpublikationen

Das Dental Vademekum. Hg.: Bundeszahnärztekammer – Arbeitsgemeinschaft der Deutschen Zahnärztekammern, Kassenzahnärztliche Bundesvereinigung, Redaktion: IDZ, 6. Ausgabe, ISBN 3-7691-4072-9, Deutscher Ärzte-Verlag, 1997

Dringliche Mundgesundheitsprobleme der Bevölkerung in der Bundesrepublik Deutschland. Zahlen – Fakten – Perspektiven. W. Micheelis, P. J. Müller, ISBN 3-924474-00-1, Selbstverlag, 1990*, Überarbeiteter Auszug aus: „Dringliche Gesundheitsprobleme der Bevölkerung in der Bundesrepublik Deutschland. Zahlen – Fakten – Perspektiven" von Weber, I., Abel, M., Altenhofen, L., Bächer, K., Berghof, B., Bergmann, K., Flatten, G., Klein, D., Micheelis, W. und Müller, P. J., Nomos-Verlagsgesellschaft Baden-Baden, 1990

Dringliche Mundgesundheitsprobleme der Bevölkerung im vereinten Deutschland. Zahlen – Fakten – Perspektiven. A. Borutta/W. Künzel/W. Micheelis/P. J. Müller, ISBN 3-924474-01-X, Selbstverlag, 1991*

Curriculum Individualprophylaxe in der vertragszahnärztlichen Versorgung. Handreichung für Referenten zur Fortbildung von Zahnärzten und zahnärztlichen Assistenzberufen. Projektleitung und Redaktion: W. Micheelis/D. Fink, Bearbeitung: J. Einwag/K.-D. Hellwege/J. Margraf-Striksrud/H. Pantke/H. P. Rosemeier/T. Schneller, Fachdidaktische Beratung von

N. Bartsch, 2. aktualisierte Aufl., ISBN 3-7691-7835-1, Deutscher Ärzte-Verlag, 1993*

Geschichte, Struktur und Kennziffer zur zahnärztlichen Versorgung in der ehemaligen DDR. Eine kommentierte Zusammenstellung verfügbarer Daten von 1949–1989. D. Bardehle, ISBN 3-924474-02-8, Selbstverlag, 1994*

Verträglichkeit von Dentallegierungen unter besonderer Berücksichtigung „alternativer" Verfahren zur Diagnostik. Abschlußbericht zum Forschungsvorhaben. Gesamtbearbeitung: H. Schwickerath, unter Mitarbeit von H. F. Kappert/J. Mau/P. Pfeiffer/G. Richter/S. Schneider/H. Schwickerath/G. K. Siebert, ISBN 3-7691-7845-9, Deutscher Ärzte-Verlag, 1998*

*Die Publikationen des Instituts sind im Fachbuchhandel erhältlich. Die mit * gekennzeichneten Bände sind direkt über das IDZ zu beziehen.*